The Cancer Unit: An Ethnography

The Cancer Unit: An Ethnography

by Carol P. Hanley Germain, R.N., Ed.D.,
Associate Professor, School of Nursing,
University of Pennsylvania

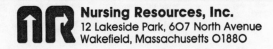
Nursing Resources, Inc.
12 Lakeside Park, 607 North Avenue
Wakefield, Massachusetts 01880

This research is dedicated to those affected by cancer and to their care givers, with the hope that the quality of care may be ever increased.

Contents

Acknowledgments

During the course of this research, I have been helped by many more individuals than I can possibly acknowledge here. I am grateful to Dr. Nobuo Shimahara, my dissertation committee chairperson from the Graduate School of Education at Rutgers University, and to Dr. Dorothy Smith and Dr. Shirley Smoyak, committee members of the College of Nursing at Rutgers University.

It requires a degree of openness and concern to share a significant part of one's life with a participant-observer. Thus, I am indebted to all those members of the anonymous hospital's nursing, medical, administrative, and departmental staffs, as well as to those patients and families who contributed their time and effort to facilitate and participate in this research.

Appreciation is extended to my professional colleagues, friends, and relatives who gave wisdom, shelter, encouragement, and prayers. Finally, I give special thanks to my husband Charley and our son "Chipper" for their love and laughter, and to my sister, Catherine Hanley, for her unswerving faith that I would indeed complete this work.

Chapter 1
Introduction

PROBLEM OF THE STUDY

An oncology unit (cancer ward) of a general hospital can be viewed as a distinct subculture whose members are affected by many variables. This ethnographic study is a descriptive analysis of such a subculture.

Societal factors that affect this subculture include attitudes toward cancer and its treatment; greater openness toward the subjects of death and dying; changing patterns of higher education; the women's liberation movement; and increasing consumer demands for participation in decision making regarding health care. Institutional factors, such as the bureaucratic control pattern in hospitals, professional-bureaucratic role conflicts, the traditional pattern of medical dominance, and the grouping of persons with various stages of cancer in a confined area, can also be expected to have an effect on the subsystem. Ideology-reality conflict within the nursing profession and the complexities of care of cancer patients may affect those members who are most consistently present in the subculture—the nurses. Additionally, the individual psychologic variables of the many actors who directly participate in the subculture (patients, nurses, doctors, families, and other hospital department members) give greater complexity to the scene.

Research attention has focused on some of these variables. However, the temporal and spatial convergence of all these and other factors in the subculture of an oncology unit makes it essential to study them in a holistic manner. A substantive study using the ethnographic approach allows us to view the situation in its total context rather than through isolated variables.

Specific Focus

The principal goal of the study was an ethnographic description of a community hospital adult oncology unit as a subculture. This included the effect of physical, physiologic, and psychologic conditions and crises of cancer patients on the intensity and extensity of social relations among nurses, doctors, administrators, patients, families, and others on the ward and in related hospital areas. The field study was carried out from May 1976 to May 1977 on a 23-bed oncology unit in a 550-bed urban, community general hospital, the Charles Hospital (a pseudonym).

Specific attention was given to the various roles that nurses play in this subculture, the problems and stresses they face in this setting, their ways of coping with these problems, and some observed consequences of their socially patterned adaptive behavior.

Assumptions

1. A hospital is a sociocultural institution that affects the behavior of people who make it up.
2. An oncology unit in a community general hospital is a unique sub-culture that can be conceptualized as a system of social relations definable in sociological and anthropological terms.
3. Such a system has a formal and an informal structure, with a set of norms and expectations, values and beliefs that regulates the behavior of its members.
4. Such a system of social relations can be studied in depth by focusing intensively upon the culture over a long period of time.
5. The research unit selected "typifies" adult oncology nursing units in community general hospitals; thus the results of such research can be generalized.

GENERAL BACKGROUND AND REVIEW OF THE LITERATURE

The following five topics provide background for the study: conflicting hierarchies in the hospital system; intraprofessional issues of nursing; cancer as an illness requiring hospital care; dying and death; and ethnographic studies of hospitals.

Conflicting Hierarchies in the Hospital System

In today's complex American society, supplying essential services to people requires highly developed sociocultural systems with role differentiation. Systems for the delivery of health services perform a critical function in maintaining the society by maintaining a level of general health that permits opportunity for other systems to achieve maximal accomplishment of their objectives.

Social institutions, organized to meet specific human problems and needs, are made up of groups of people governed by implicit or explicit cultural rules or by established expectations of behavior in a network of organized social relations. One such institution, the community general hospital, has been developed by modern society for the care of its sick members.

A hospital has been defined as a complex and specialized problem-solving system that utilizes an organizational structure as its major mechanism [1]. In the hospital organizational structure, there are two distinct hierarchies: the administrative bureaucracy and the medical profession. Ultimate legal authority and responsibility are vested in a board of trustees or directors. Registered nurses are responsible for the greatest amount of activity directly related to the physiologic and psychosocial care of patients. However, nurses, most of whom are women, must respond to the male-dominated administrative bureaucracy as well as to the male-dominated medical hierarchy, whose members exercise nearly exclusive control over medical policies but are attached to the hospital organization as individual entrepreneurs.

In addition to being responsible for the larger part of patient care, the nursing service department has also traditionally been the repository of maintenance and coordinative functions in the hospital system by virtue of the fact that nursing is the only professional group that is present twenty-four hours a day. However, nurses are generally excluded from major administrative and medical decision-making structures.

Ashley, reporting on the historical development of hospitals and hospital schools of nursing in American society, asserts that physicians and hospital administrators have consistently sought to economize in hospitals by exploiting women. This sexist oppression has resulted in a limitation of nursing's function, with consequent detriment to the care of patients [2].

Intraprofessional Issues

Although nursing has little power, it is numerically the largest of the health care professions. In a 1972 inventory, there were 1,127,657 registered nurses in the United States holding licenses to practice. Of these, 98.7 percent were women. Of the total, 11.8 percent had completed the baccalaureate degree in nursing, and 2.2 percent the baccalaureate degree in other fields. Sixty-nine percent of all registered nurses were employed, and 64 percent of the total were employed in hospitals [3].

Presently there are three pathways to registered nurse licensure: the two- or three-year hospital diploma school program; the community or junior college program, usually two years, which awards the associate degree; and the generic baccalaureate program, usually four years, which culminates in a bachelor's degree with a nursing major. While there are differences in the goals and expected outcomes of these programs, there has been little or no distinction in the kind of work done by graduates of the different programs at the hospital staff nurse level [4]. This situation has given rise to the expression, "A nurse is a nurse is a nurse."

Today the nursing profession is concerned with developing greater professional self-esteem and autonomy and with moving away from institutionalized self-definitions of inferiority [5]. Recent changes in the Nurse Practice Acts of several states give legal support to independent functions of the nurse. The preparation of nurses has changed from a task-oriented, procedural orientation to a biophysical and psychosocial science base, with a problem-solving approach to patient care, including assessment, diagnosis of nursing care needs, goal-setting, intervention, and evaluation. The literature gives considerable evidence of application of this "nursing process" [6].

The traditional hospital diploma school curriculum deliberately emphasized learning role-specific behaviors and values to be used in the ward work of the associated hospital. In marked contrast, baccalaureate nursing programs today are moving toward an integrated, process-oriented curriculum. The integrative rather than the additive character of learning is stressed, with a focus on learning how to learn and nurse (process) as well as on acquiring knowledge and skills. The purpose of this approach is to prepare nurses to discover and utilize concepts and principles that can be generalized across care environments, clinical areas, and age groups. However, when a neophyte baccalaureate nurse takes a hospital staff nurse position, she is subject to what Kramer calls "reality shock," because of the disparity between the skills and values she has been taught and those that are rewarded in the work situation [7].

The American Nurses Association, the national professional organization for registered nurses, had approximately 196,024 members as of December 31, 1974 [8]. In 1965 the ANA took the position that nursing education should be in the mainstream of American higher education rather than in the tradition of the hospital school. It stated that not all nurses need to be professional practitioners (with at least baccalaureate level nursing preparation), but that professionals should be responsible for all nursing care, giving leadership and direction to technical-level nurses, whose basic preparation would be through the associate degree [9]. This position had a divisive effect on the profession, since many nurses felt that it downgraded their hospital-based training. Hospital-school graduates were particularly fearful that the traditional state license designation of registered "professional" nurse would be eliminated, and they would receive the lesser status of "technical" nurse.

More recently the New York State Nurses' Association has drawn up a resolution to revise the Nurse Practice Act of that state so that by 1985 a baccalaureate degree in nursing would be required for licensure as a registered professional nurse, and an associate degree in nursing would be required for licensure as a practical nurse. This proposal for two levels of licensure has generated considerable intraprofessional debate. An alternative proposal calls for not changing the present licensure for registered nurses and practical nurses but creating a new designation for those with baccalaureate degrees in nursing, who would be licensed as professionally independent nurses (INs) [10].

Nursing today is moving in the direction of meeting Flexner's criteria of a profession [11]. Many nurses with preparation in a clinical specialty view themselves as peers of physicians and other health professionals (although this view is often not reciprocal). Other indicators of professionalism in nursing are an emphasis on building its own body of knowledge through nursing research, refining its literature, and providing doctoral programs with a nursing major.

However, in the researcher's relatively extensive experience as a teacher of hospital-employed registered nurses in university-sponsored continuing education courses in nursing, it was apparent that many nurses were not prepared for the transition from a task-oriented, physician-dominated mode of hospital practice to a professionally autonomous one. Many nurses, especially older ones, find security in the status quo and are resistant to change. They cite lack of time and lack of staff as their reasons for not carrying out systematic planning, execution, and evaluation of nursing regimes. Such factors as tradition, ritualism, obeisance, institutional constraints, and lack of skill in problem solving or in writing nursing orders are rarely mentioned as reasons. The traditionally oriented nurse often views proponents of scientific-based collaborative nursing practice as "ivory tower idealists," who are far removed from the realities of everyday life on the ward.

The functions of nursing have been classified from various perspectives. In a legal framework, Lesnik and Anderson have identified seven functional areas of professional nursing, based upon existing legislative and judicial decisions. Only one of these seven functions is identified as dependent: "the application and the execution of legal orders of physicians concerning treatments and medications with an understanding of cause and effect thereof" [12].

This one "dependent" function raises the critical issue of professional autonomy, defined by Friedson to mean "the quality or state of being independent, free, and self-directing," which in the professions refers mostly to control over the content and terms of one's work [13]. In the health field, Friedson considers only medicine and dentistry as truly autonomous, since they have the authority to direct and evaluate the work of others without being subject to formal direction and evaluation by them.

In contrast, however, some nursing leaders assert that there are no dependent functions in nursing, only independent or collaborative ones. Dr. Martha Rogers states:

> Nursing exists to serve society, and nurses are directly responsible to the people they purport to serve. The nursing profession does not exist to serve the ends of any other profession, nor does one profession delegate anything to another profession. Each profession must determine its own boundaries within the context of social need. As a learned profession, nursing has no dependent functions but like other professions, has many collaborative functions that are indispensable to providing society with a higher order of service than any one profession can offer [14].

Several sociologists, however, disagree. Etzioni classifies nursing as a "semiprofession" along with teaching and social work, although he concedes that nurses are "less typical" semiprofessionals because their decisions have an effect on life and death [15].

Simpson notes that the semiprofessions are dominated by bureaucratic control rather than control by autonomous groups of colleagues. She cites the hospital nursing service as an example. There is great emphasis on hierarchical rank, with administrative tasks replacing core tasks, that is, patient care, and greater status is accorded those who are "promoted" away from direct patient care. She also notes that all the forces for bureaucratic control of the semiprofessions are strengthened by their predominantly female composition:

> The public is less willing to grant autonomy to women than to men. A woman's primary attachment is to the family role. . . . they are less likely than men to develop colleague reference group orientations; they are culturally socialized to defer to men and hence are more willing to accept bureaucratic controls than genuinely professional status, and they do not base their career choice on scholarly attraction to the intellectual content of their intended work [16].

Katz views the nurse not as a professional but as a "nonscientific, care-minded person," who accepts a low place in the hospital's status hierarchy. She not only agrees to help the physician in his scientific tasks, but also helps overcome inadequacies in the scientific method of practicing medicine by keeping knowledge about errors, ambiguities, and uncertainties from reaching patients and their families.

> If she were a full-fledged professional peer of the physician, she could, conceivably, take a more active moral stand against mistakes in medical treatment. But, as it stands, she is chiefly a sponge and a buffer. . . . The destruction of the caste system so that nurses can make their full contribution will take much imaginative effort [17].

Friedson contends that in the hospital organization, where medicine is the dominant profession, "It is as true for the worker as for the patient that the professionally organized division of labor has pathologies similar to those resulting from bureaucracy" [18]. The physician is protected by organized autonomy and is not bound by rules from outside his profession, though his performance can set up barriers to communication and result in evasion and in reduction of the client or worker to an object. "Professional dominance is the analytical key to the present inadequacy of the health services" [19].

In the hospital, the doctor's written order is virtually the only formal mechanism by which doctors influence nurses, and the nurses are formally obligated to carry out these written orders. The informal ways in which doctors influence nurses have been described by a psychiatrist using a "game" model and calling the type of interaction a transactional neurosis. The nurse is taught to make significant recommendations to the doctor but in such a way as to make it appear that he initiated them. Since most nurses are women, elements of the game reinforce the stereotyped roles of male dominance and female passivity [20].

Historically, the militaristic style of hospital nursing schools fostered the view that the physician had infinitely more knowledge than the nurse. As part of her enculturation, the student learned subservient mannerisms and gestures of deference to physicians. The result is that nurses socialized to the profession in this manner have a fear of independent action that is most marked when relating to physicians. This is illustrated by the research in which twenty-one of twenty-two nurses were prepared to give a patient an excessive dose of an unknown drug ordered by an unknown male telephone caller who claimed to be a physician. They were intercepted before harm was done to a patient [21]. In their study of hospitalized patients, Duff and Hollingshead found that physicians assigned to nurses the role of assistant [22].

Byerly states that hospital-employed registered nurses are affected by a number of pressures, including multiplicity and ambiguity of authority, vulnerability to criticism, problems in aligning and reconciling therapeutic and managerial functions, status disparity, and the need to respond psychologically to these and other pressures in socially and culturally accepted ways [23].

Leininger identifies two current subcultures of nursing, an old one and a new, emerging one, which are differentiated by major cultural patterns or themes. The traditional culture is marked by qualities of other-directedness, self-sacrifice, dedication, deference to paternalistic figures such as physicians and hospital administrators, and dependence upon persons in authority. The traditionally enculturated nurse is passive, compliant, nonquestioning, a doer rather than a thinker, practical, intuitive, and socially insecure. Her practice emphasizes physical aspects and expressive-giving care. She relies on symbolic objects, such as the uniform, cap, and pin, as important media to communicate her identity as a professional. Her manner is dignified, self-controlled, and passive.

In contrast, nurses of the new culture are concerned with sharing power and decision making with physicians and hospital administrators, being independent in practice, meeting their own needs and goals, and using collective bargaining rights to negotiate both economic security and practice issues. They resist authoritarian norms, place less emphasis on doing and more on thinking, and fuse expressive (nurturant) and instrumental (technical) role behaviors. They are also described as less concerned with symbolic crutches, more self-expressive, candid, open to their limitations, and socially more secure [24]. The women's liberation movement has been a major force in the new socialization of nurses toward more assertive behavior.

Cancer as an Illness Requiring Hospital Care

In the United States today, cancer ranks second as the cause of death for males and females in both the white and nonwhite populations. It was estimated that in 1977, 690,000 persons would be diagnosed for the first time as having cancer, and 385,000, or one person every one and one-half minutes, would die of the disease. On the other hand, there are three million Americans alive today who have a history of cancer. Two million of these are without evidence of the disease at least five years after diagnosis and initial treatment ("cured") [25]. On the average, cancer will strike about two out of every three families.

With rare exception, cancer is a chronic disease. Patients may require hospitalization for diagnosis; for various forms of initial treatment; for treatment of metastases (spread to secondary sites), recurrences, complications, or advanced disease; and for care in the terminal phase.

Generally, the diagnosis of cancer carries with it threats of death (or at least curtailed life), pain, disfigurement, odor, and various social and economic losses. Feder found that in persons with malignant disease, being hurt or abandoned was of more concern than death per se [26].

Data collected in the Third National Cancer Survey indicated that 1.3 million cancer patients are under hospital care each year. Sixty-one percent of a sample of 3,151 cancer patients required one hospital admission during the two-year period following diagnosis; the average number of admissions was 1.7 per patient. In this survey a typical hospital stay for a cancer patient lasted an average of sixteen days and cost about $1,400 per stay [27]. Given the rapidly increasing cost of hospital care, this figure would be much higher today.

There has been a marked increase in the modalities of cancer treatment over the past decade. Radical surgical techniques, radiotherapy with X-rays or radioactive materials, chemotherapy, hormones, and immunotherapy have increased longevity for cancer patients. Regional cancer treatment centers, particularly for megavoltage radiotherapy, have been established in community general hospitals as well as in metropolitan research centers. The medical subspecialties of radiation oncology and medical and gynecologic oncology have been developed. Today those who are active in the field of cancer care try to present a positive perspective—that cancer is a chronic disease to be lived with rather than a "death sentence" [28].

Many cancer patients receive adjunctive therapies on an ambulatory basis. When hospitalization is required, however, there is a tendency to group cancer patients on one unit because of the specialized nature of the treatment. This puts increased demands on nurses, since the nursing of cancer patients is highly demanding in both the technical and expressive roles. Strauss, Fagerhaugh, and Glaser note that in hospitals, distinguishing patterns of ward work and organization do exist. The work or the sentimental order of the ward itself can be affected by various events on the ward [29], and as Caudill noted, by events in the larger organization as well [30]. An oncology unit is an example of this.

In reference to the care of cancer patients, Benoliel and Crowley state:

> Part of a well established tradition, only recently begun to be questioned, is the idea that somehow, somewhere in the education of the nurse and the physician, something magic happens to free them from personal reaction to pain, mutilation, disfigurement, offensive odors, sights or sounds, while at the same time preserving, and in fact, nurturing an exquisite sense of sensitivity and compassion. In fact, personal reactions to unrelieved pain, disfigurement, and mutilation are a real strain in providing care to such patients. Furthermore, the patients whose pains are not completely relieved and the patients whose illnesses cannot be cured are, in some sense, an affront to care and treatment—a reminder of man's finiteness and limited capacity to control his environment [31].

A physician has stated that "in the sense that vastly more sophisticated treatment is today available, the life of the cancer patient may well depend on the caliber of nursing care that is available to the patient" [32]. Yet a cancer nursing specialist states that "cancer nursing is wide open for lack of nurses" [33]. This is attributed to the complex nursing care needs of these patients and their families—physiologic and psychologic crises are not uncommon.

Though there is a massive amount of published research on cancer, most of it is basic research into the etiology of cancer or its treatment. Cancer nursing literature largely deals with reports of nursing care procedures or programs for cancer patients in hospices, hospitals, or homes. Ayers and others note that research in cancer nursing is in its infancy; a survey of the literature from 1963 to 1973 yielded only thirty-three cancer nursing studies, dealing with cancer screening programs, psychosocial needs of patients and the reactions of physicians and nurses to the diagnosis of cancer, patients' physical and rehabilitative needs, and surveys of learning needs of personnel [34].

Pienschke found that patients had greater confidence in their physicians and nurses and perceived nurses as more effective when there was an open approach to the diagnosis of cancer on a cancer unit. Physicians tended to be open with the diagnosis but guarded with regard to prognosis [35].

Parsons, in a descriptive study of intermediate-stage terminally ill cancer patients in noncrisis periods in their homes, found that despite the severity of the disease, these patients had minimal physical problems and were able to discuss their feelings about living with cancer and impending death. Their helping agents were mostly family members [36]. Hampe's research showed that the spouses of terminally ill cancer patients had eight needs related to anticipatory grief [37].

Evaluation of an inservice education research project, designed to teach nurses to interact therapeutically with dying patients and their families, did not strongly support the efficacy of the program [38]. More recently, oncology nursing specialty groups have given greater emphasis to the promulgation of nursing research.

Dying and Death

Death is a social fact, real and inescapable, though the research of Glaser and Strauss, Quint, and others has indicated that until recently death has been a taboo topic in American society [39, 40]. Once a natural event that took place in the home with natural supports, the process of dying has become an American social problem. Factors that complicate the process include technological developments that change the statistical frequencies from early death toward increased longevity but with chronic disease, and new therapies that may lengthen the time between the onset of a fatal illness and death. Medical training so emphasizes healing and prolonging life that the dying patient comes to represent a failure, and his death offends the healing-oriented physician [41]. Research has indicated that nurses are likely to avoid contacts with dying patients [42].

Like other societies, American society has developed institutionalized means for minimizing the social disruption brought about by individual deaths. Hospitals, where most Americans die, classify and route dead patients in an efficient manner, though this bureaucratization of death often has negative consequences for the dying and for the survivors. With hospitalization of the dying, patients and families must adjust to new personnel, new treatment locations, financial strain, interpersonal conflict, and increased emotional suffering on the part of the patient. Glaser and Strauss note:

Much, if not most, non-technical conduct toward, and in the presence of, dying patients and their families is profoundly influenced by common sense assumptions, essentially untouched by professional or even rational considerations or by current advancement in social-psychological knowledge [43].

The individual and collective denial of death has been explained by Freud and many others as a psychologic defense mechanism necessary to deal with the overwhelming anxiety produced by the threat of death. As Berger and Luckman note: ". . . death also posits the most terrifying threat to the taken-for-granted realities of everyday life" [44].

Over the past decade there has been a growing interest in the science of death (thanatology) and a greater research interest in the process of dying. Sudnow studied the handling of death and the dead in a county hospital whose clients were charity patients and in a private hospital. He found that hospitals are organized to hide the facts of dying and death from patients and visitors. For example, when death was imminent the dying patient was moved to a private room [45].

In another hospital study, Glaser and Strauss studied the management of information about dying, with the central issue being "awareness of dying." They distinguished four awareness contexts: the situation in which the patient does not recognize his impending death though everyone else does (closed awareness); the situation in which the patient suspects what the others know and therefore attempts to confirm or invalidate his suspicion (suspected awareness); the situation in which each party defines the patient as dying but pretends that the other has not done so (mutual pretense awareness); and the most favorable situation for reducing isolation and depersonalization, one in which personnel and patient seem to be aware that he is dying and act on this awareness quite openly (open awareness) [46].

From her experience with several hundred terminally ill hospitalized patients, Elisabeth Kübler-Ross constructed a typification of the five stages of the dying process. These adaptational strategies or stages are: (1) denial and isolation ("no, not me"); (2) anger ("why me?"); (3) bargaining ("if you give me one more year, I'll go to church"); (4) depression ("yes, it's me"); and (5) acceptance [47]. The stages may overlap, and a patient may go back and forth between stages. Without needed emotional support, some may become fixated in one stage and not reach the final stage of acceptance.

Kübler-Ross indicates that when the dying patient is given the opportunity to communicate his sentiments, frustrations, or expectations about dying, he enlarges his competence to accept death. She says, "These patients have taught us . . . that they are all aware of the seriousness of their illness whether they are told or not" [48]. She views the "open awareness" context as optimal for most patients. Significantly, Quint's research on dying patients showed that many nurses in practice were taught as students how to take care of the dying patient's body but had little preparation for interacting with the dying person. Medical school curricula showed a similar gap [49].

Now in the developmental stage in the United States, a new social institution, the hospice, has as its major goal providing supportive care for dying patients, their families, and friends. The hospice concept includes care at home as well as in an independent facility, or more recently, in hospital units. Patterned after the work of Cicely Saunders in Great Britain, the hospice concept stresses each patient's individuality and his continued accessibility to family and friends [50].

Ethnographic Studies

Ethnographies, or factual descriptions of the way of life of a specific group of people, are integral to the work of social and cultural anthropologists. Field study, a principal anthropological method of studying people, permits gathering data about a designated group's lifestyle within its natural setting and sociocultural context.

Field studies have been done in psychiatric hospitals, partly because as closed systems with "captive" populations they are somewhat easier to study than the more open system of a general hospital. Goffman and Caudill did field studies of inpatient psychiatric settings [51, 52]. Strauss and colleagues did a comparative field study of two private and public mental hospitals and discussed the influence of hospital structure on nurses' role behavior [53]. Rosenhan used the participant-observer technique in a psychiatric hospital investigation [54].

Few ethnographies of general hospitals or their nursing units have been found in a search of the literature, though the technique of participant observation has been used in studies conducted in general hospitals by Jackson, Duff and Hollingshead, Millman, and others, and in nursing homes by Henry [55-58]. Coser studied the role of the patient in a general hospital ward, investigating how the social organization of the ward affected patients' adjustment [59]. Fox studied a metabolic research unit with emphasis on the role of the research physician and the patients [60].

Buckingham used the technique of participant observation to compare the effectiveness of a palliative care unit for terminally ill patients with that of care of the dying on a general ward [61]. However, Buckingham, a medical anthropologist, became a pseudopatient, and his true identity remained unknown for the duration of the study, which raises the serious ethical issue of informed consent by research subjects [62, 63].

Byerly did an ethnography of a medical-surgical nursing unit in a general hospital, emphasizing the role behavior of registered nurses in the system. The need for ethnographic studies of general hospital units has been stated by Byerly, Leininger, and others [64, 65].

RESEARCH METHODOLOGY

Gaining Entrance

The researcher's interest in doing an anthropological study in a hospital arose from the complaints and frustrations expressed by nurses in a continuing education course called "The Nursing Process," which she taught for a state university. The course essentially presented a problem-solving approach to nursing practice, and the students, many of whom were nurses at hospitals in the area, expressed considerable resistance and skepticism about the change from task-oriented nursing to a scientific approach. Some comments expressed frustration at the idea of institutional change, "That could never happen here." Resistance was noted in comments such as, "If that's the way nursing is going, then I'm glad I'm ready to retire." Ideology-reality conflict was reflected by the statement, "Whoever writes those books doesn't know what it's like in the real world." However, the researcher had some questions about the extent to which nurses contributed to maintaining the status quo.

One section of the course was taught at the Charles Hospital, which provided classroom space adjacent to its medical-nursing library. For the majority of the twenty enrollees, it was their first semester-length nursing course in over twenty years. Most were unaccustomed to using the library, a fact validated by the librarian, who stated that nursing students used it, but registered nurses employed in the hospital rarely did. The hospital administration paid the nurses' tuition for the course, which was held from two to four in the afternoon so that the nursing personnel enrolled from the day and evening shifts could attend as part of their paid work day and also avoid a trip back to the inner city in the evening. Most of the course participants were head nurses or team leaders.

During the year before the course was given at Charles, a new director of nursing had been appointed. Because of her announced level of preparation, the researcher believed she might be receptive to the idea of a nurse doing research in the hospital sociocultural system. The researcher initially contacted the director of nursing in an exploratory discussion about a field study. The researcher presented several ideas about anthropological studies in hospitals and the nature of descriptive research (which she later found were interpreted by the director as studies of ethnicity and patient care). When the researcher presented a formal proposal, the nursing director was somewhat hesitant about a field study of the hospital sociocultural system; she stated that the researcher would have to discuss the idea with the hospital administrator, who could not schedule an appointment until six weeks later.

In his well-appointed executive office, the administrator posed some pertinent questions, such as, "What is anthropology?" and, "What does an anthropologist do in a hospital?" but gave support to the idea of a field study. Although the researcher was originally interested in studying a general medical-surgical unit, the oncology unit, a specialized unit for the care of patients with cancer, was offered. One major reason stated for the limited choice of units was that the general medical-surgical units were preparing for the arrival of medical students from a nearby university, and some turmoil in the organization of medical care was anticipated. The director of nursing also suggested that the limited number of admitting physicians and the lower patient census of the Oncology Unit would make the study more manageable for the researcher.

The administrator impressed the researcher with his knowledge about field studies in hospitals and the degree of freedom necessary for a researcher in the participant-observer role. He acknowledged that there would be some obstacles, such as physician resistance, but declared his full support of the project.

The director of nursing and the nursing supervisor of the Oncologic Unit (who had taken the researcher's course) were also receptive to the proposal, which involved a minimum of three, three-hour visits per week for one year. Permission to take photographs was denied before the researcher posed the question. Further stipulations included approval of the proposal by the medical director of the Oncology Unit; a written, legal contract between the university and Charles Hospital, exempting the hospital from liability for any harm to patients if the researcher participated negligently in nursing care activities, and exempting Charles Hospital from any liability for personal harm or injury to the researcher; proof of professional licensure; and proof of personal, professional liability insurance. The researcher was to wear a white lab coat and a temporary employee's identification badge, the latter for security reasons.

After these conditions were met, the researcher met with the director of nursing, the supervisor, and the head nurse of the unit to clarify for the head nurse what the researcher's role on the unit would be, primarily with respect to nursing care. Neither the head nurse nor the nursing staff had read the proposal but had approved the study after hearing it explained by the supervisor, who was the liaison person for the study. Because the researcher was a nurse, the staff initially tended to interpret the term "participant observation" as limited to traditional staff nurse functions rather than to anthropological research. The supervisor's comment, "Well, Carol, we'll put you on the time sheet," was an example of this. The primacy of the research role had to be clarified so that nursing staff and physicians, in particular, did not have unreasonable role expectations of the researcher. Her participation in traditional nursing functions was selective, determined by the goals of the research. She needed to be free from the constraints of an assignment so that she could wander, observe, write notes, or participate in meetings that would not usually be accessible to a member of the staff.

Throughout the research year, the writer felt accepted, for the most part, as Junker states: "more as participant ('good friend') than as observer ('snooping stranger')" [66].

Research Techniques

Participant observation was the major research technique, with extensive field notes providing a record of much of the data collection.

The role of participant-observer in field work can take several forms. Junker describes four different types: complete participant, participant as observer, observer as participant, and complete observer. Junker notes, however, that the practicing field worker oscillates through the range of the four types. In this study, the researcher did assume all of the roles at various times, but "observer as participant" was her primary role.

> This is the role in which the observer's activities as such are made publicly known at the onset, are more or less publicly sponsored by people in the situation studied and are intentionally not kept under wraps. The role may provide access to a wide range of information, and even secrets may be given to the fieldworker when he becomes known for keeping them, as well as guarding confidential information. In this role the social scientist might conceivably achieve maximum freedom to gather information but only at the price of accepting maximum constraints upon his reporting [67].

In addition to data from the Oncology Unit, pertinent data were gathered in related departments of the Charles Hospital and at professional and social gatherings of employees held at other locations. To help the researcher gain a better perspective of the care of cancer patients, the unit's medical director arranged an informative observational experience with "well" cancer patients in his office.

In the data-gathering process, all information was treated confidentially. Anonymity in reporting was assured and is provided through the use of pseudonyms for the institution and its location, as well as for all persons referred to in any way.

While the researcher became well known during the research year to those involved with the study unit as well as to many others in the institution, no general announcement was made of her presence or purpose in the hospital. Whether or not to make such an announcement had been left to the discretion of the hospital administrator and the director of nursing.

When it was appropriate for the researcher to introduce herself, she told interviewees that she was a graduate student doing a study of the Oncology Unit as a "small society" and that she was also a nurse. She then answered any questions posed about the research or her role, and also explained that the data would be handled in a confidential manner.

While most introductions were at the personal level, the researcher did meet with some groups to explain and answer questions about the research and their willingness to participate; these groups included the nursing staff of the unit, nurses in an orientation program, nursing students from Charles Hospital's School of Nursing, professional and lay persons attending family conferences, a staff meeting of oncologists, and informal groups in the cafeteria and coffee shop.

After the first few days in the field, as the researcher became better known and accepted by the nursing staff, their introduction of her to other hospital staff members changed from a rather awkward "Carol's doing her doctoral in anthropology," to one that reflected their perception of the field of anthropology. For example, the head nurse remarked, "Carol's here to study our savage tribe"; and one of the staff nurses commented, "Carol's doing an appropriate study. This place is getting more like a zoo every day."

Feedback from the staff on the researcher's entry into and role in the subculture was obtained unsolicited as well as solicited on several occasions. For example, the supervisor said, "We told Mrs. Bowman [the director of nursing] that Carol's here, but nobody acts as if she's around." Several months into the study the head nurse remarked, "I can't get over how the staff has accepted you. It's like you're not even an outsider. They pay no attention to you." It is recognized that these comments do not necessarily represent the whole range of reactions to the researcher's presence.

A second major source of data was interviews, structured and unstructured, individual and group. To obtain baseline data, the researcher made appointments for interviews with individual members of the nursing staff, the three oncologists, regular support staff to the unit (public health coordinator, social worker, chaplain), two hospital administrators, the director of nursing, and the director of inservice education. Numerous opportunities for informal interviews with these members were also utilized. Family conferences, nursing staff conferences, change-of-shift reports, and nursing staff support sessions afforded opportunities for interviewing those groups. Unstructured interviews often took the form of impromptu discussions at various locations in the hospital. They were sometimes focused but often serendipitous.

When permission was granted, individual and group interviews were tape recorded and later transcribed. In the interests of validity, raw data (direct quotes of members of the subculture) have been used extensively in this report of the research. In many ways, the actors tell their own story very well. Material quoted was taken from tape recordings or from brief notes taken unobtrusively during interviews and completed shortly thereafter. Since it is virtually impossible to record verbatim quotes during a nontaped interview, quotation marks in this report indicate that the material enclosed is as accurate a record of what was said as is possible under rapid note-taking conditions. The summary, conclusions and recommendations in Chapter 7 are solely the researcher's.

In the course of a three-hour period in the field, the researcher would stop several times to write down notes; detailed descriptions of incidents and conversations were written down as soon as possible after they occurred to limit distortion. When it was feasible, she asked individuals or groups about their perceptions of events and their feelings about them shortly after the event. Field notes were typed as soon as possible, and data were roughly categorized concurrently. Seven months additional time was required for writing the first full draft of the manuscript.

A three-hour field visit usually had at least one specific focus, such as observing an individual or group in their daily activities, making rounds with the head nurse or doctors, attending a conference or change-of-shift report, conducting a formal interview, or talking with a patient or family. There was ample time to follow up on ongoing situations or to get involved with new developments. Since the researcher was free to wander, she did not keep a strict schedule, except for appointments, but moved to whatever location she judged valuable for data collection. It was made clear to staff that their individual participation was voluntary and that patients' care needs should not be jeopardized to accommodate research goals. For that reason, staff were sometimes unable to keep appointments or were unable to discuss their observations promptly after an event. Broken appointments were rescheduled, and the time was used for other research pursuits. Often the reason for a broken appointment, such as a crisis on the ward or a nurse's involvement in a patient-family situation, afforded a ready opportunity for further data collection. The staff were often voluntarily helpful in pointing out events they thought would be valuable for the research. Physicians sometimes called the researcher's attention to patients who they thought were interesting because of medical phenomena or family stress.

Subjective Adequacy

Bruyn cites several rules of experiential evidence that are useful for gauging the accuracy of findings in participant observation studies. These rules deal with the key concepts of time, place, social circumstance, language, intimacy, and consensus [68].

Time. Twelve months of active participant observation on the research unit was necessary in order to learn about and be accepted by the people in the subculture; to witness and participate in a wide variety of the system's activities; to follow through on certain issues to their conclusions; and to find out how members of the subculture viewed their roles and explained their behavior as individuals and members of the collectivity. The researcher maintained personal and telephone contact with key informants for a subsequent five-month period during data analysis for further clarification and follow-up on how issues were resolved. The pattern of three, three-hour visits each week was generally maintained. Hours were varied so that all times of the twenty-four-hour day, seven-day week were sampled. Most of the observations took place during the most active period, the day shift (7:00 A.M. to 3:00 P.M.), but one month each was spent on the evening and night shifts.

Place. Most of the field study took place on the Oncology Unit. Additional locations of data gathering included small interviewing rooms; the Admissions Office; an inservice education classroom; a hospital tour; the lounge of the Self-Care Unit one floor below the research unit, where family conferences were held; the offices of other hospital department members, such as the administrator, nursing service director, social worker, finance officer, medical records librarian, and public health nursing coordinator; other hospital clinical departments, such as Radiation Therapy; the archives room of the hospital library; and the hospital school of nursing.

Social circumstance. The researcher sometimes had meals or coffee breaks with the nursing or medical staff in the employees' cafeteria or coffee shop so that she could meet with individuals or small groups in a more relaxed environment. The researcher also attended the hospital's annual fund-raising fair, a retirement tea for one of the nurses' aides, and a Christmas party for the nursing staff, which was paid for each year by one of the oncologists (Dr. Long) and held in the afternoon in the lounge of the Self-Care Unit. A national cancer nursing conference gave the researcher some opportunity for socializing with the head nurse, a nurse from the Radiation Therapy Department, and a nurse who worked in the office of one of the oncologists. The researcher also attended a local American Cancer Society conference, where she was able to hear a talk given by one of the oncologists and confer with nursing staff members away from the research environment.

Language. This term includes all those forms of communication that are significant in the society being studied such as words, tone of voice, facial expressions, gestures, pointed silences, or slang expressions. Before entering the field, the researcher knew the basic medical terminology and hospital slang, which was necessary in order to study the hospital system and subsystems, and she readily learned the terms and slang expressions peculiar to the oncology subculture. Other forms of communication used as data for this study included the patients' charts, employees' newsletters, local newspapers, administrative memoranda, letters to the nursing staff from patients and families, hospital archives, formal and informal interviews with individuals or groups, and conferences of various types.

Intimacy. The success of a researcher's entry into a culture can be assessed by the degree to which members share matters that are not usually open to outsiders. During this study, the researcher was invited to join some nursing and medical conferences and social occasions that were closed to outgroup members. A number of individuals voluntarily sought the researcher and shared information and/or feelings not shared openly with other members of the subculture.

The unit's nursing supervisor, the designated liaison between the researcher and the institution, was open, available, and helpful. If asked for something beyond her jurisdiction, she would generally indicate an access barrier by stating that she would have to seek clearance at an upper level of the hierarchy. The researcher was not given permission to attend head nurses' or supervisors' meetings. Individual staff evaluation conferences were not accessible for reasons of privacy. With individuals and groups, the researcher was sensitive to cues concerning limits and did not push beyond them.

In the reporting, the only limitation was imposed by the supervisor and the head nurse and involved the identity of the individual who was found to be engaged in deviant social behavior on the unit over the course of the year. Those circumstances will become clear to the reader further on in the study.

Consensus. A conscious effort was made to verify data by seeking direct confirmation of specific observations, events, and issues from the individuals involved. By posing the same questions to different informants, the researcher sought to determine if there was general agreement on the phenomenon in question.

Midway in the research year, the researcher was ready to leave for a short vacation just as several critical events on the unit were about to converge. In order to have a record of the continuity of events, she employed as an "assistant" a staff member who had seemed objective in her appraisal of events on the unit thus far. The assistant kept a log on the days she worked and wrote it up as a summary at the end of the day. Though it was recognized that her job responsibilities limited her mobility and her objectivity, nevertheless her observations were validated by the charge nurse when the researcher returned to the unit.

The charge nurse's first remark was, "Have I got news for you!" She then talked for twenty minutes, particularly about the unit's "most difficult patient ever," Jim Jason. The head nurse and supervisor later volunteered their perspectives on events that had occurred in the researcher's absence, basically validating the assistant's observations.

Formal structures have both public and private aspects, and access to the private aspects has been thought to be difficult for outsiders. According to Goffman, officials in institutions are concerned with "impression management." He states:

We often find a division into back region, where the performance of a routine is prepared, and front region, where the performance is presented. Access to these regions is controlled in order to prevent the audience from seeing backstage and to prevent outsiders from coming into a performance that is not addressed to them. Among members of the team, we find that familiarity prevails, solidarity is likely to develop, and that secrets that could give the show away are shared and kept [69].

Data in this study are presented as a valid expression of individuals' and staff's perception of their current social circumstances. Some of the data may seem remarkably "back region"; no attempt has been made to assess the motivations of individuals who provided such data.

Bias. It was sometimes difficult to select phenomena for data collection because of the numbers of patients, staff, rooms, departments, activities, and situations. A single participant-observer had to be selective in her involvement, which raises the question of bias. Schwartz and Schwartz state, "One's frame of reference influences selections one makes from the phenomena and determines how and what is observed." These researchers also assume "that the observer can and does know what his biases are and that knowing what they are, he can, by specifying them, prevent distortion of his observations" [70].

Quint notes that when field work is used as a research method, the participant-observer becomes the instrument of the research, since the data are collected and analyzed by a human observer. She emphasizes that it is necessary "to use one's inner conflicts and biases as an essential part of the data being collected and analyzed" [71].

In the data collection, the researcher made a determined effort to attend to the varying elements that would contribute to a holistic view of life on the cancer ward. In the analysis and reporting of data, she emphasized separation of the usual from the unusual, the commonplace from the idiosyncratic, and concentrated on those phenomena found repeatedly to be significant.

The Nurse as Anthropologist

Since the research goal was to discover, describe, and explain the nature of the subculture as it was given, the researcher's general policy was non-intervention, so as to disrupt ongoing social processes as little as possible and to minimize the change induced by her presence. As a nurse well socialized into the professional role, however, the researcher often had to resist the practice role of "doing" for the research role of observing how things got done. This aroused guilt feelings at times, as when she had to leave the unit, knowing it was short-staffed with many unmet patient care needs. At these times the researcher kept reminding herself to take a long-range view of the potential benefits of this research rather than the short-range view of providing care that others were there to give.

At times, the researcher felt compelled to intervene, as when she had information that might change the staff's view of a patient's situation. In the environment of a cancer unit, it was next to impossible simply to observe or listen. Unpredictable and urgent patient situations sometimes compelled action, such as positioning a basin for vomitus, helping a patient quickly to the bathroom, helping someone to cough up a mucus plug, or supporting an emotionally distressed patient or family member. Valentine states, "Nor do we . . . feel it is always possible to avoid intervention, especially in participant ethnography which requires that one constantly interact with the community not just as observer but also as fellow citizen" [72].

The assumed nursing role seemed natural, for it allowed the researcher to ease in and out of patient care situations. When the researcher was with a patient or responded to a patient's call light when staff were unable to respond as quickly, her usual course was to meet immediate needs for personal, supportive, safety, comfort, or technical care, when these needs were obvious or requested. Some needs could be met without staff assistance, but many such actions or observations had to be reported to the nurse in charge of the patient, or to another member of the nursing staff. Some requests were beyond the physical capacity of a single person. An early observation was that a strong back is a major prerequisite for nursing on an oncology unit. The researcher commonly listened to patients or families or simply gave a helping hand, such as a cup of tea in the middle of the night to a sleepless patient.

When a group was discussing controversial issues about which the researcher had strong opinions, however, she felt comfortable remaining an observer rather than an active participant in the discussion. She did state her opinion if it was directly solicited. The researcher also contributed at nursing staff conferences or family conferences when she believed that certain significant input was not forthcoming from the group, but her participation was low-keyed. The researcher found herself getting involved in staff education, mostly by supplying articles that she thought would be helpful but which the staff were not likely to obtain elsewhere, and by calling their attention to continuing education programs that would not normally be announced to them.

There were times when the research role conflicted with other values, such as a patient's privacy, or when certain aspects of staff behavior on medical rounds were professionally embarrassing, which necessitated leaving the scene or stepping aside so as not to be identified with the group. One time on rounds the group went to see Mr. Reardon, who was very ill and weak. Two nurses were supporting him on a bedpan while he was expelling an enema. Dr. Long pulled up a chair opposite Mr. Reardon's flexed knees, opened the chart, and proceeded to ask him questions about his medical orders, to the accompaniment of expelled gas and liquid. The researcher stepped outside.

Inevitably, as a researcher talks openly with patients, families, or members of the staff in the data-gathering process and listens to their views, complaints, regrets, hopes, or fears, some change occurs, however minimal, that would not have been induced if she were an unseen observer. At times the anthropologist-researcher was also nurse, teacher, counselor, friend, confidante, or helper. It is the researcher's view that these roles enhanced data collection in this subculture.

The researcher was familiar with and participated in many hospital organizations. As a clinical instructor of nursing students, she had learned to orient herself rapidly to many types of nursing units in a large number of hospitals. She had had nursing experiences with relatives and friends with terminal and arrested cancer. The language of the subculture was not foreign to her.

Because of these experiences, the researcher was able to avoid the magnitude of "culture shock" that a nonnurse anthropologist might have experienced in this setting. Nevertheless, she did experience an initial shock and a continuing, though lesser, emotional reaction, as she witnessed the continual, collective destruction wrought by a savage force—the disease of cancer—in the patients, the families, and some of the staff.

While the traditional role of the research scientist, as Bruyn points out, is:

> that of a neutral observer who remains unmoved, unchanged, and untouched in his examination of phenomena, the role of the participant observer requires sharing the sentiments of people in social situations; as a consequence he himself is changed as well as changing to some degree the situation in which he is a paticipant [73].

Finally, the researcher wishes to reemphasize that pseudonyms have been used throughout the study. Also, she has purposefully used titles or first names of individuals according to the way in which these people were addressed, in order to reflect the subculture's nuances and forms of social interaction.

REFERENCES

1. Georgopoulos, B. The hospital system and nursing: some basic problems and issues. *Nurs. Forum,* 5(3): 8, 1966.
2. Ashley, J. A. *Hospitals, Paternalism, and the Role of the Nurse.* New York: Teachers College Press, 1976, p. ix.
3. American Nurses' Association. *Facts About Nursing 76-77.* Kansas City: ANA, 1977, pp. 1-3.
4. Hogstel, M. Associate degree and baccalaureate graduates: do they function differently? *Am. J. Nurs.,* 77: 1598, 1977.
5. Benoliel, J. Q. Scholarship—a woman's perspective. *Image,* 7 (2): 26, 1975.
6. Browning, M. (comp.) *The Nursing Process in Practice.* New York: American Journal of Nursing, 1974.

7. Kramer, M. *Reality Shock*. St. Louis: C. V. Mosby, 1974.
8. American Nurses' Association, 1976, p. 53.
9. American Nurses' Association. Position on education for nursing. *Am. J. Nurs.*, 65: 106, 1965.
10. McGriff, E., and Simms, L. Two New York nurses debate the NYSNA 1985 proposal. *Am. J. Nurs.*, 76: 930, 1976.
11. Flexner, A. Is social work a profession? *School and Society*, 1: 901, 1915.
12. Lesnik, M., and Anderson, B. *Nursing Practice and the Law*. Philadelphia: J. B. Lippincott, 1955, pp. 258-279.
13. Friedson, E. *Professional Dominance*. New York: Atherton, 1970, p. 136.
14. Rogers, M. Nursing: to be or not to be. *Nurs. Outlook*, 20: 44, 1972.
15. Etzioni, A. (Ed.). *The Semi-Professions and Their Organization*. New York: Free Press, 1969, p. xiv.
16. Simpson, I. Women and Bureaucracy in the Semi-Professions. In Etzioni, A. (Ed.), 1969, p. 197.
17. Katz, F. Nurses. in Etzioni, A. (Ed.), 1969, p. 71.
18. Friedson, E., 1970, p. 145.
19. Friedson, E., 1970, p. 145.
20. Stein, L. The doctor-nurse game. *Arch. Gen. Psychiatry*, 16: 699, 1967.
21. Hofling, C. et al. An experimental study in nurse-physician relationships. *J. Nervous and Mental Dis.*, 143: 171, 1966.
22. Duff, R., and Hollingshead, A. *Sickness and Society*. New York: Harper & Row, 1968, p. 23.
23. Byerly, E. Registered Nurse Role Behavior in the Hospital Sociocultural System: A Systems Approach. Ph.D. dissertation, University of Washington, 1970, pp. 7-8.
24. Leininger, M. The Traditional Culture of Nursing and the Emerging New One. Chapter 5 in *Nursing and Anthropology: Two Worlds to Blend*. New York: John Wiley & Sons, 1970, pp. 63-87.
25. American Cancer Society. *1977 Cancer Facts and Figures*. New York: ACS, 1976, pp. 3-4.
26. Feder, S. Attitudes of Patients with Advanced Malignancy. In *Death and Dying: Attitudes of Patient and Doctor*. New York: Group for the Advancement of Psychiatry, 1965, pp. 614-622.
27. U.S. Department of Health, Education and Welfare. *Cancer Rates and Risks* (2nd ed.). Washington: DHEW publication No. (NIH) 75-691, 1974, p. 3.
28. American Cancer Society. *Proceedings of the National Conference on Cancer Nursing*. New York: ACS, 1974, passim.
29. Strauss, A., Fagerhaugh, S., and Glaser, B. Pain: an organization-work-interactional perspective. *Nurs. Outlook*, 22: 560, 1974.
30. Caudill, W. *The Psychiatric Hospital as a Small Society*. Cambridge: Harvard University Press, 1958, pp. 3-28; 317-344.
31. Benoliel, J., and Crowley, D. The Patient in Pain: New Concepts. In *Proceedings . . .*, 1974, p. 74.
32. James, A. What is New in Prevention and Control. In *Proceedings . . .*, 1974, p. 17.
33. Hilkemeyer, R. Cancer Nursing: the State of the Art. In *Proceedings . . .*, 1974, p. 7.
34. Ayers, R., Baker, V., and Padilla, G. Research in Cancer Nursing. In *Proceedings . . .*, 1974, p. 25.
35. Pienschke, D. Guardedness or openness on the cancer unit. *Nurs. Research*, 22: 484, 1973.
36. Parsons, J. A descriptive study of intermediate stage terminally ill cancer patients at home. *Nurs. Digest*, 5: 1, 1977.
37. Hampe, S. Needs of grieving spouses in a hospital setting. *Nurs. Res.* 24: 113-120, 1975.
38. Padilla, G., Baker, V., and Dolan, V. *Interacting with Dying Patients: An Inter-*

Hospital Nursing Research and Nursing Education Project. Duarte, Cal.: City of Hope Medical Center, 1975.

39. Glaser, B., and Strauss, A. *Awareness of Dying.* Chicago: Aldine, 1965, p. 3.
40. Quint, J. *The Nurse and the Dying Patient.* New York: Macmillan, 1967, p. 1.
41. Kaspar, A. The Doctor and Death. In Feifel, H. (Ed.), *The Meaning of Death.* New York: McGraw-Hill, 1959, p. 259.
42. Quint, J. The threat of death: some consequences for patients and nurses. *Nurs. Forum,* 8(3): 286, 1969.
43. Glaser, B., and Strauss, A. *Time for Dying.* Chicago: Aldine, 1968, pp. ix, 284.
44. Berger, P., and Luckman, T. *The Social Construction of Reality.* New York: Doubleday, 1967, p. 101.
45. Sudnow, D. *Passing On: The Social Organization of Dying.* Englewood Cliffs, N.J.: Prentice-Hall, 1967, pp. 65-66.
46. Glasser, B., and Strauss, A., *Awareness of Dying,* 1965.
47. Kübler-Ross, E. *On Death and Dying.* New York: Macmillan, 1969.
48. Kübler-Ross, E., 1969, p. 233.
49. Quint, J., 1967, p. xiii.
50. Paige, R., and Looney, J. Hospice care for the adult. *Am. J. Nurs.,* 77: 1812, 1977.
51. Goffman, E. *Asylums.* Chicago: Aldine, 1961.
52. Caudill, W., 1958.
53. Strauss, A. et al. *Psychiatric Ideologies and Institutions.* Glencoe, Ill.: Free Press, 1964.
54. Rosenhan, D. On being sane in insane places. *Science,* 176: 250, 365, 1973.
55. Jackson, B. An experience in participant observation. *Nurs. Outlook,* 23: 552, 1975.
56. Duff, R., and Hollingshead, A., 1968.
57. Millman, M. *The Unkindest Cut.* New York: William Morrow, 1977.
57. Henry, J. Human Obsolescence. Part 3 in *Culture Against Man.* New York: Random House, 1963, p. 391.
59. Coser, R. *Life in the Ward.* East Lansing, Mich.: Michigan State University Press, 1962.
60. Fox, R. *Experiment Perilous.* New York: Free Press, 1959.
61. Buckingham, R. W. et al. Living with the dying; use of technique of participant observation. *Canad. Med. Assoc. J.,* 115: 1211-1215, 1976.
62. American Nurses' Association. *Human Rights Guidelines for Nurses in Clinical and Other Research.* Kansas City: ANA, 1975.
63. Armiger, Sister B. Ethics of nursing research: profile, principles, perspective. *Nurs. Research,* 26: 330, 1977.
64. Byerly, E., 1970, p. 262.
65. Leininger, M., 1970, p. 164.
66. Junker, B. *Field Work: An Introduction to the Social Sciences.* Chicago: University of Chicago Press, 1960, p. 38.
67. Junker, B., 1960, p. 38.
68. Bruyn, S. *The Human Perspective in Sociology.* Englewood Cliffs, N.J.: Prentice-Hall, 1966, pp. 207-218.
69. Goffman, E. *The Presentation of Self in Everyday Life.* New York: Doubleday, 1959, p. 238.
70. Schwartz, M., and Schwartz, C. Problems in participant observation. *Am. J. Sociology,* 60: 352, 1955.
71. Quint, J. Role models and the professional nurse identity. *J. Nurs. Educ.,* 6(2): 11-16, 1968.
72. Valentine, C. Models and muddles concerning culture and inequality: a reply to critics. *Harvard Educational Review,* 42: 105, 1972.
73. Bruyn, S., 1966, p. 14.

Chapter 2
The Charles Hospital
and Its Administration

HISTORY OF THE HOSPITAL AND SCHOOL OF NURSING

The Charles Hospital was a 550-bed, JCAH-accredited, hundred-year-old general hospital located in the city of Lafayette, which was also the county seat. During its centennial celebration, a year prior to the start of the research, the hospital's name had been changed to the Charles Medical Center to reflect its new status as a major affiliate of the state medical school; but it shall be referred to here as the Charles Hospital.

The conglomerate of twelve hospital buildings took up a full block of the inner city. Surrounding the hospital was evidence of advanced urban decay—dilapidated, mostly unoccupied two- and three-story row houses with broken windows, sagging porches, and garbage- and glass-covered sidewalks and gutters.

Charles Hospital was the brainchild and financial legacy of a close-knit family of unmarried siblings whose ancestors had settled in the area in the late 1600s, seven generations earlier. The land donated for the hospital had been owned by the family since the early 1700s. In the late nineteenth century the surviving siblings conveyed the grounds to a legally constituted hospital corporation. The hospital was originally named after the city, Lafayette; but the nine-man Board of Managers voted to change the name to that of the donor family prior to the hospital's dedication.

Charles Hospital was to be a free hospital; its act of incorporation declared that its purpose was "to afford gratuitous medical and surgical aid, advice, remedies and care to such invalid and needy persons as, under the rules and by-laws of said corporation shall be entitled to the same." Though the archives do not state a religious affiliation, the founding fathers of the hospital belonged to a small religious group, and retiring members of the Board of Managers were usually replaced by familial descendants.

In the 1870s, when sheep still roamed the hospital grounds, the city of

Lafayette was in its growing phase. When the hospital finally opened in the 1800s, the population of the city was around 55,000, and with the arrival of European immigrants, it continued to grow. Various sections of the city became ethnic ghettos of Poles, Irish, and Italians. By mid-twentieth century the population of the prosperous city was about 125,000.

After that the national phenomenon of middle- and upper-class white flight to suburbia affected Lafayette. There was an influx of blacks, Puerto Ricans, and other Spanish-surnamed groups, and in the late 1960s a wave of urban racial unrest touched the city. Store after store on the major shopping street closed down. By the early 1970s, sections of the city looked as if they had been bombed out. The 1970 census revealed a population of about 105,000, of which about 40 percent were blacks; 12 percent, Spanish-surnamed; and 48 percent, Caucasians. Eighty-five percent of the city's population was on welfare.

The rise and decline of the city closely paralleled that of the Charles Hospital. Although the original building was completed in the 1870s, the hospital could not open until ten years later, when sufficient operating funds became available. Since all patients were to receive free care, the hospital's income was expected to come from interest on invested funds from the original legacy as well as from endowments and contributions. Early annual reports of the Board of Managers listed the names of donors and their monetary or material contributions. Sums of twenty-five and fifty cents were recorded, as well as contributions of "old linen" and five dollars' "conscience money." Other listings, a decade later, included two baked hams, an ear trumpet, and an air cushion.

Originally, the patient units were large open wards. As hospitalization insurance became more common and the demand for semiprivate rooms increased, the wards were gradually reconstructed. Service buildings and departments and patient care units were added over the years.

In Charles Hospital's first year, 290 patients were admitted, and the endowment income covered 100 percent of patient care costs. By the mid-thirties, when over 8,000 patients were admitted, only 8 percent of the cost was provided by endowment income.

Bylaws of the Board of Managers and Rules for the Government of Charles Hospital were adopted when the hospital was incorporated. Sections of the rules were specific to certain personnel, such as the matron, the chief nurse, the medical residents, and nurses. Among the rules relating to nurses was: "Nurses are expected to remain standing when speaking to the Physicians and while they are in the wards, and to conform strictly to the uniform worn in the hospital."

Patients, too, had rules to observe. For example:

Patients are forbidden—
    to quarrel

to use profane or indecent language, to express immoral or infidel sentiments; to have any book, pamphlet, or newspaper of an immoral or indecent nature
to talk loud, sing, or whistle
to lie in or upon the bed without being undressed.

Patients who disregard or disobey any of the above rules shall be liable to be
discharged by the Visiting Committee, or in their absence, by the Resident
Physician.

The Visiting Committee, two members of the Board of Managers, made
rounds once a week and made dispositions regarding patients who viola-
ted the rules.

A school of nursing was part of the structure of the Charles Hospital
almost from its opening. One early annual report stated:

Recognizing the necessity for trained and skillful nurses to execute with
loyalty and obedience the directions of the physician in the sick-room, the
attending staff of the Charles Hospital resolved to supply this deficiency by
organizing a training school for nurses. In 1889, The Lafayette Training
School for Nurses, which subsequently became the State Training School
for Nurses, was organized at The Charles Hospital under the care of the
attending staff, and was chartered during the following month. Since then,
the system of nursing has been revolutionized . . . ; the monthly nurse has
been relegated to the past; aseptic and antiseptic methods of nurse practice,
and what to observe and record in the progress of the disease, have been
inculcated.

The one-year course was lengthened to two years a few years later and
to three years a decade after that. A "didactic and demonstrative course
of instruction" was given. Lectures in medical nursing, surgical nursing,
gynecological nursing, obstetrical nursing, and contagious nursing were
taught by doctors, and their names and subjects published in the annual
report. The early curriculum also included lessons in "Invalid Cookery,"
"Massage," and "Swedish Movements." One of the first nurses to
graduate was elected "demonstrator." Over the first twenty years of its
existence, graduating classes varied in size from one to twelve women.
The annual reports of this early period listed all of the graduates of the
school by year of graduation and indicated their present employment or
other status. The reports include comments such as: "Pupil nurses
receive the benefit of lectures by the attending staff, lectures on and
instruction in massage in addition to the practical training on the
wards."

In the early 1890s, the state legislature passed an act empowering any
training school for nurses that offered specific courses to confer the
degree of Medical and Surgical Nurse (M.S.N.). For an uncertain length
of time, the Charles School of Nursing conferred such a degree on graduates who passed its examinations. However, since the creation of a state

board of nursing, the school has been approved to award only a diploma. The school has never applied for accreditation by the National League for Nursing, the official accrediting agency for basic nursing programs. A spokesperson for the school said that the administration would not appropriate the accreditation fee, believing the process to be "too costly" and the league's efforts "coercive."

A nurses' home was constructed at the turn of the century, and since the school continued to grow, a dormitory and classroom building was added on the corner of the property about twenty-five years later. This building connected to the original nurses' home by an outdoor walkway at the second-floor level. In the late 1960s this was converted to hospital use, and new classrooms and living space were obtained for the student nurses in a commercial building a block away. The school still graduates about thirty nurses annually. The current director has been with the school for more than twenty-five years.

CURRENT DEVELOPMENTS

While the city around it decayed, the hospital's legacy also decayed, the patient load increased, and the hospital came close to bankruptcy. Over the years, it had expanded the scope of its services to the point that it became known as one of the region's chief hospitals. But the conservative spending policy of its founders had resulted in neglect of the physical plant. In the early seventies the Board accepted the plans of the administrator, Mr. Smith, for a rebuilding program on the same site. Subsequent to this decision, the Charles' horizons expanded when it agreed to affiliate with the state medical school. A few years later, ground was broken for a new, ten-story, five-hundred bed hospital, and a schedule was made to demolish its deteriorated old buildings.

Because federal and state legislation and various accrediting agencies had greatly increased the workload of the Board of Managers, Mr. Smith recommended that it be expanded and that the corporate structure be changed, creating the new position of president-chief executive officer. The person filling this position was to be responsible for community and medical school relations and development, while the executive vice-president-administrator, Mr. Smith, was to remain responsible for the day-to-day operation of the hospital. Positions on the board were designated for three physicians plus the president of the medical staff; no other group, such as nursing, was specifically represented on the board. About midway through its research year, the hospital announced the appointment of Dr. Eric Jones, a physician with background in management and medical school organization, as the new Charles president.

Dr. Jones told the researcher about some Charles Hospital history that was not available in the archives. He stated that the basic structure of the original Board of Managers remained until after World War II, when the board hired an administrator. The goal of the first administrator, who had been a bank loan officer, was to make Charles the biggest and least expensive hospital in the region. He didn't replace buildings or take care of basic structural needs, and he had almost no functional relationship to the medical staff; in fact, the relationship was almost entirely an adversary one.

During the first administrator's tenure, the Board was composed of second- and third-generation descendants of the founding family and the original Board. A separate Women's Board, largely made up of wives of the Board of Managers, carried out fund-raising activities and held an annual picnic on the grounds. When the first administrator got into a squabble with the Women's Board, they complained to the Board of Managers, and the administrator was fired. He walked into the office of his assistant, Mr. Smith, and said, "Everything you need to run this hospital is in this file cabinet. I'm retiring," and he left.

Mr. Smith, whose previous experience had been at a thirty-bed hospital in the rural South, had been at Charles for only two years at that point. According to Dr. Jones, Smith was:

> A lovely, warm, friendly guy, but not a decision maker. He avoided change and decision making by saying "no." While he kept the per diem down— the rate here a few years ago was $55 while every other hospital in the state was $102 to $105—he did it by letting his own assets go. The place was filthy and falling apart. While there was no great stress or drive for quality care, I suppose people did the job fairly well. But resistance to change here is incredible. Tremendous changes were taking place elsewhere but not here. Eight years ago the hospital was virtually bankrupt.

Dr. Jones explained that in the late 1960s, when the need for a new hospital building became evident, some of the medical staff tried to donate suburban land so they could move from the inner city. However, the businessmen on the board did not want the hospital to leave the city, both because of the original charter and the fact that the suburban areas had sufficient hospitals. Then half of the medical staff invested their own money and hired a building corporation to erect a new hospital on the suburban land. When most of these doctors left the active admitting staff at Charles, admissions dropped off about 50 percent, although they later came back up.

Soon after he was hired, Dr. Jones' presence became known to hospital staff through an announcement in the Charles newsletter and various posted notices. One memo stated that in order to get to know the hospital and its staff better, Dr. Jones was going to make "management rounds." The nursing supervisor accompanied him and a management group on a tour of a teaching unit for medical students. Dr. Jones' response to this tour was described as sheer exasperation; the unit was so confused and chaotic that he never ventured out on rounds again. He described it to one of the staff as "like Times Square on New Year's Eve."

Dr. Jones' appointment created anxiety in the hospital hierarchy, because the staff did not know what effect the changes being made in organizational structure, such as the personnel and housekeeping departments, would have on them or on the work order of the hospital. A supervisor remarked, "This place is in a state of organizational crisis, but nobody knows it except the nurses."

Subsequent to Dr. Jones' arrival, when the researcher had seen Mr. Smith in the cafeteria, he had pleasantly inquired about her progress with data collection and expressed his concern that she was getting what she needed.

Midway in the research year, Mr. Smith's resignation was announced in the Charles newsletter, which was a shock to a great many people. The accompanying article stated that Mr. Smith had held the administrator's position for the previous six years. The article described the progress that the institution had made during his tenure; a new power plant and a 600-car parking garage were built; cardiac catheterization, respiratory therapy, radiation therapy, and nuclear medicine departments were initially or more fully established; long-range building plans were adopted; and ground was broken and construction started for the new hospital.

Shortly after reading the newsletter, the researcher met Mr. Smith in the hall. When she commented that she hadn't anticipated his resignation, Mr. Smith responded: "I didn't, either. It was my own idea to expand the Board of Managers and secure a president whose major concern would be community affairs and development of medical education; but, in effect, I talked myself out of a job."

Mr. Smith said the situation had become increasingly difficult after Dr. Jones' arrival. The assistant administrators had difficulty because they had to report to "two masters," himself and Dr. Jones. Early on, Mr. Smith lost control of the budget when Dr. Jones made this his exclusive domain, and gradually, he was stripped of his other powers and responsibilities. When he took some time off to reflect on his situation, he kept coming to the same conclusion—it wouldn't work out; it was impossible to be in a powerless position after having been the chief executive officer for six years. Upon his return he had negotiated with Dr. Jones to have a small office and a secretary for six months. His major occupation became job hunting.

Since this conversation was taking place in a hallway, the researcher told Mr. Smith that she would make an appointment with his secretary to meet with him and discuss the situation further. Mr. Smith said that no appointment was necessary—he had nothing else to do. "I have nothing but time. I don't keep calendars. I have no need for them. I'll be glad to see you and talk about anything you'd like."

The researcher asked Mr. Smith whether he thought there would be some major changes at Charles because of the medical school affiliation. Mr. Smith said, "There is a real risk when the emphasis is on medical education that patient care will suffer. And care is important in a community hospital." He stated that the reason a union had lost in a recent employee election was that he had spoken with the employees. He continued:

> Eighty percent of the lower-echelon employees were born in this hospital or had relatives cared for here. I said to them, "How can you deal with the union philosophy that says you should walk away from your own relatives who are sick?"

The word "family" was frequently used by and about Mr. Smith. For example, the article in the employee newspaper announcing his resignation stated that "Mr. Smith is a fair but firm administrator who cherishes his Charles family." A security guard said, "Mr. Smith is just like one of us, he often sits with us in the cafeteria during lunch." Another employee commented, "He's always a good sport who never hesitated to appear in holiday skits or lead the Christmas caroling."

A few days later, the researcher went to Mr. Smith's office. No longer located in the executive suite, his office was at the end of a ward in the oldest patient care section of the hospital, with a desk for himself and for a secretary. Describing his last few months as administrator, Mr. Smith stated:

> I took over a failing, deteriorating hospital. The medical staff didn't agree that we should stay in Lafayette, but now they think it's a good move. They want a medical school but are not one hundred percent in favor of full-time faculty or heads of departments.

> Priorities changed this year after the building program started. The medical school became the number one priorty. It was not the board's decision to move me out of the job. I've had lots of regrets from board members. Jones will run a one-man show. I can't agree with everything he's doing. I can compromise my principles just so far.

An interview with Dr. Jones, published in a major area newspaper about six months after his arrival, emphasized the grave nature of the hospital's financial ills; it had lost half a million dollars the previous year. Dr. Jones blamed much of the problem on state health department regulations that controlled the amount Charles could charge insurance carriers and Medicaid for patient care. The health department allowed $130 per day, but the hospital's cost was $143 daily. Additionally, Charles claimed it lost two million dollars that year caring for the medically indigent patients (uninsured low-income people who make too much money to qualify for Medicare or Medicaid), who made up 9 percent of its census.

The state claimed that Charles' problems resulted from poor financial management. The vice-president for finance claimed that until five years earlier, the Charles had run a very cheap operation. Instead of replacing equipment when it broke down, the board repaired and repaired and repaired. They let the century-old building deteriorate to the point that it was about to fall down. At that time, hospitals were allowed to set their own insurance reimbursement rates. Since the Charles Hospital wasn't spending much, its costs stayed low. However, in the early seventies, when the board committed itself to a spending program, the state limited the amount that hospitals could be reimbursed. Also the Charles was about to start paying the principal and interest on a $38,000,000 construction loan for the new building.

The day after these comments were published, was a particularly hectic one on the Oncology Unit. In the late morning, Mildred, the part-time registered nurse in charge, got a call from the hospital's fund-raiser advising her that she was delinquent in her pledge to the building fund. In the middle of trying to cope with a number of hassles, she explained to the man that she had not pledged to give on a regular basis but would contribute when she could. After she hung up, she griped to the people at the desk. The clerk asked if the others had seen the article in the paper. "How come," she asked, "that Dr. Jones makes $65,000 per year while Mr. Smith only made about $30,000?" At that moment, the fund-raiser appeared on the unit with some papers and asked for Mildred. She let him know, loudly and clearly, that she had no intention of repeating her initial donation on a regular basis. He retreated with papers in hand.

When the researcher went to see Dr. Jones several months after his arrival, she asked him about his impressions of the small society since he had become its new chief.

> It's a mess, a total, complete, absolute mess. I killed three cockroaches the day I came in for my interview. There are no systems of internal control—no way of checking on things. One day when I first came, I saw 40 to 50 charge slips in a wastepaper basket. We buy 50 percent more food than is needed. There is no security. We are losing 40 to 50 percent through theft and overbuying. You can tell war stories all year long.

Dr. Jones stated that he was in the process of changing the entire finance department and that a new senior vice-president for finance had been appointed. He added that he had had windows cleaned, rooms painted, and had bought two hundred new suites of furniture. Another change was that no patient in the emergency room was to be asked about his method of payment before being examined. "Everybody thinks I'm crazy. We may lose money, but we make friends," said Dr. Jones.

In the late spring, while talking to the four members of the Nursing

Inservice Education Department, the researcher asked how the change in administration had affected their department.

The two younger instructors commented:

A lot of positive things are coming from it. There's somebody to go to who will give good reasons for approving or disapproving.

We never had an outgoing decision maker like him before.

We've gone from a family to a business, which is fine.

He definitely wants to improve patient care. He got windows cleaned, paper towels in the bathrooms. But physicians aren't ready for him.

Change is for the better. The place wasn't organized two and a half years ago. There were no paper towels or wastebaskets in patients' rooms. The scene was very lax all the way from nursing practice on up. Nursing only had a few procedures written down.

The director of the department, who had been silent but perturbed-looking, said, "Mr. Smith is not to blame for all of this."

An instructor replied, "He's one of the friendliest people, but his casual manner also carried over to business practice. You need a business mind. Here, I don't need a family, I have one at home. I need quality control and more production."

Another stated:

Dealing with the individual idiosyncrasies of doctors is a major problem here, but headway is being made. Doctors through the years thought nurses were handmaidens. Now we are intelligent handmaidens. Just recently a doctor wanted to lecture to the student nurses on what the role of the head nurse should be, and he was invited.

The director of the department appeared uncomfortable and asked the researcher: "Who is going to read this material?" The nature of the study and the use of pseudonyms were reemphasized.

The researcher also asked the director of nursing, Mrs. Bowman, how the change in top-level administration had affected nursing. "It hasn't affected nursing too much except in the case of integrated progress notes," she replied. That change had been initiated by this memo from Dr. Jones:

In light of recent JCAH and state health department recommendations, effective in one month, all progress notes will be integrated in one section.

The tabbed section marked PROGRESS NOTES will be the only section available for physicians and all supporting staff departments to record their progress notes.

At Charles, as is traditional in most hospitals, doctors recorded daily progress notes in one section of the patient's chart. Unit nurses recorded their notes in a separate section called "Nurses' Notes." Other nurses, such as the public health coordinator, and other departments, such as social services or physical therapy, recorded on separate consultation sheets. Nurses, over the years, often complained that doctors didn't bother to read nurses' notes, and doctors retorted that there was nothing of value to read.

After Dr. Jones' memo about progress notes, the nursing Inservice Education Department prepared nurses for the change by holding classes on the essentials of a nursing progress note. Nurses' reactions were mixed Some favored the idea; others were concerned about the greater exposure their notes would receive and their ability to meet higher expectations.

The doctors' response, however, was immediate and organized resistance, but their objections to Dr. Jones' dictum, voiced through representatives, were overruled.

Despite the lack of social and professional communication among the three main admitting physicians on the Oncology Unit, they were united in their opposition to integrated notes. One, Dr. Long, vented his irritation by circling nurses' spelling errors or by writing notes in the margin. For example, one nurse wrote that a patient complained of constipation. He wrote, "Why didn't you give her an enema?"

With time and experience, nurses' notes improved, and there were fewer objections. In fact, some of the doctors' written comments were positive. For example, when Rita, a registered nurse, described an increase in sensory and motor loss in a patient's lower extremities, Dr. Long wrote, "Above noted and appreciated." Dr. Fisher wrote "good comment" next to Rita's recording of a statement by a patient who had been referred from another hospital: "I know I have cancer, but my doctor didn't tell me that."

When the researcher asked Dr. Jones about the issue of integrated progress notes three months after the policy went into effect, he replied:

> Next month I'll probably withdraw the proposal for a short period. The medical staff is very threatened, and this is another threat. They know their care needs to be better; they know we are going to hire full-time department chairmen. However, the joint commission and the state will undoubtedly request it again. In six months it will probably be law anyway. We will have lost only a few months, but on the second try there will be less resistance and we will start with some experience. Nurses have not performed well at it; they have not tried to use it in a sophisticated way.

Before he was able to implement plans to withdraw the proposal, Dr. Jones became ill and took a recuperative leave, returning fully recovered two months later. Subsequently, the medical staff appealed the issue of integrated progress notes to the Board of Managers, who overruled Dr. Jones's mandate. Thus, after six months of experience, the use of integrated progress notes ceased. One of the nursing supervisors described the doctors' reaction as, "It was like 'we beat you', but we [nurses] were never in a contest with them."

The researcher also asked Dr. Jones about his views on the future of the Charles School of Nursing. He said:

> Contrary to what your professional associations (ANA and NLN) advocate, I don't think most nurses should be baccalaureate degree nurses. I see two categories of nurses: career nurses, and you may not like the expression, chauvinistic nurses. These latter use nursing for whatever their personal reasons are. To me the A.D. [Associate Degree] program is the answer. In this area there are not enough A.D. programs. At the moment, simply because it's convenient, the diploma school serves a purpose.

> The social milieu has not changed enough for most nurses not to be concerned with being a housewife and with motherhood. As they learn to manage rearing a family with two employed parents, the scene will change. Where I came from, over 90 percent of the working nurses were younger than twenty-five or older than thirty-five. They drop out for ten years. We can't change those values until society changes them.

THE NURSING DEPARTMENT

Organization

Under the old administrative organization, the director of nursing also had the title of assistant administrator, and had a direct-line relationship to the administrator. Under the new organizational structure, the director of nursing's title was vice-president for nursing affairs. She was part of an Operations Group that also included two senior vice-presidents, one for medical affairs and one for administrative affairs, who was responsible for the day-to-day operations of the hospital. The vice-president for nursing affairs reported to the senior vice-president for administrative affairs. One of the staff members stated, "There are really two layers of vice-presidents. Mrs. Bowman reports to Harry Anthony, who is a horse's ass."

In a line relationship to the director of nursing were the departments of Nursing Service, Nursing Education (including the school of nursing and in-service education), Nursing Quality of Care, Special Tests, and Public Health Nursing. The director of nursing was occasionally seen on the Oncology Unit escorting a prospective staff member. On one occasion she checked on narcotics record signatures, looked at the Kardex nursing care plans, and commented to the staff at the desk that "nursing care plans should relate to the patient's chart and vice versa."

In the Nursing Department there was also an associate director who worked during the day and five day supervisors who related to either the director or the associate director. The director of nursing met separately each week with the supervisors and the head nurses, primarily to discuss policy and procedural changes and implementation. Each head nurse was expected to communicate information from these meetings to the nursing staff of her unit. The director of nursing stated that she did not believe in mass meetings of different levels of the nursing staff.

The supervisors were first-line managers, who, according to the director, had overall responsibility for the daily management of several units, including responsibility for "environment, staff, patient care, evaluations, and disciplinary actions." The director viewed some supervisors as "more aggressive in decision making than others." Supervisors got extra vacation and compensatory time, and they managed their own time. They took turns "covering the house" on weekends.

Nurses at Charles did not always go through nursing administrative channels to solve their problems. In November, when a staff shortage on the Oncology Unit became critical and help did not seem forthcoming, the head nurse spoke to Dr. Fisher about it. He replied, "If the staffing problem is not solved, we will close beds and admit patients to the general wards of the hospital. This is a specialty unit, and if it doesn't have enough nurses, we can't admit patients." Another staff nurse, discussing the traumatic events during a staff shortage the year before, said, "A year ago Dr. Fisher did put in for overtime for us."

It was a hospital policy, reinforced by the supervisor, that nurses' aides did not get overtime, that they were supposed to leave work on time. But an aide said, "If the nurses are giving the report and we answer a patient's light, sometimes we have to completely change the bed and bathe the patient. How are we supposed to walk out at three-thirty?" What upset the very conscientious and hard-working aides was that if they clocked in late because of car failure or some other unpredictable event, their paycheck was docked, regardless of how much overtime they had worked.

Within the last few years, head nurses at Charles Hospital had been promoted to the managerial level. According to a key informant, this status was granted so that the head nurses would be ineligible to be part of a collective bargaining unit. There were no collective bargaining units at Charles, but the informant said:

> We have no unions, but the administration proceeds as if we do, so as to discourage employees from organizing. Employees are given the opportunity to bid on job vacancies before they are publicly advertised, and this tends to keep outside influences from moving in. Head nurses are supposed to get certain management privileges, like not working every other weekend as the staff nurses are required to do. But they can only exercise that privilege if their units are covered. When you don't have enough staff, that doesn't mean anything. Head nurses are supposed to have flexibility in their hours—to come in at night for example, to troubleshoot. But they're in in the morning before the rest of the staff, and they never get off on time anyway.

One member of the school of nursing faculty was on the membership committee for the district group of the state nurses' association, which is a constituent of the American Nurses' Association. In the spring, a program to attract new ANA members was to be held at another hospital in the city. Permission to post the announcement of the meeting outside the nursing office at Charles was denied because one of the seven topics to be discussed was "Economic and General Welfare," which is the collective bargaining arm of ANA. Another topic was "Standards of Nursing Practice and Continuing Education." The hospital that had offered its facilities for the meeting withdrew the offer also.

The wages for staff-level registered nurses at Charles were $5.40 per hour plus an "experience factor," $4.20 for licensed practical nurses, and $3.60 for aides. Since the head nurses were considered part of management, their salary level was not publicized.

Members of the Nursing Department worked an eight-hour day on one of three shifts: 7:00 A.M. to 3:30 P.M., 3:00 P.M. to 11:30 P.M., and 11:00 P.M. to 7:00 A.M. A half hour was allowed for lunch or supper. There were no cafeteria or coffee shop services at night, but there was a food cart that sold sandwiches and beverages for a short period each night.

At Charles, supervision of the night nursing service was separate from that of the other shifts. It was impossible to tell who would be working that night from looking at the weekly time sheet at the nurses' station. The researcher was told that day supervisors controlled only the day and evening shifts and that the night supervisor made out the time sheet for all night employees, which was kept in the main nursing office. The Oncology Unit was not staffed by full-time RNs on the night shift; in the researcher's short experience on the night shift she met three part-time registered nurses who were assigned to be in charge of the unit on a per diem basis, resulting in lack of continuity of patient care. There seemed to be no logical explanation for the separateness of the night nursing service, it was just a tradition. According to the director of nursing, who had been at Charles only three years: "There is inbreeding because of the school of nursing. This is not a big problem except in effecting change. So much is tradition—not written down. It's always been."

Charles Hospital had a Nursing Council, consisting of the director and associate directors, the inservice education director, and two supervisors. Any change in or addition to nursing policies, procedures, or standard care plans had to be approved by this group. Proposed changes that involved medical aspects of care also had to be approved by the Executive Committee of the Medical Staff, made up of doctors who were present or past chiefs of service. During a nursing staff orientation session that the researcher attended, it was explained that, within the last three years, it had taken the doctors one year to agree to a particular policy change proposed by nursing. The nurses wanted to be allowed to use their judgment about whether a patient who had been given an enema should get up to go to the bathroom to expel it. Long-standing policy said that patients must expel enemas into bedpans in bed unless a written doctor's order to the contrary was given. Dr. Irwin, an orthopedist, led the opposition to this policy change, because one of his patients had gotten up to go to the bathroom to expel an enema but had accidentally expelled it on the floor, slipped in it, and broke his leg and had died later of complications. Eventually the issue was decided in the nurses' favor.

A Nursing Liaison Committee, which was chaired by a physician and consisted of other doctors, including the chief resident, and several nurses, was supposed to deal with problematic doctor-nurse relationships. However, the problems brought to the committee mostly concerned nurses and the nonattending staff, that is, interns, residents, and medical students. Physician attendance at meetings was described as "poor." The physician in charge, Dr. Martha White, was described by one of the nurses on the committee as "terrific." The researcher asked if she thought that this quality had something to do with the fact that the physician was a woman; she was told, "Dr. White was a nurse before she went to medical school."

Formal institutional norms or rules were contained in policy and procedure manuals. Because certain of these norms concerning administration of medications, a process which was highly ritualized by the Inservice Education Department, were dysfunctional for the Oncology Unit, they were often ignored by the staff. Other rules from the Nursing Policy Manual included:

> Permission must be obtained from the charge nurse before any toenails can be cut.
> Difficult toenails must be referred to the physician.
> Toenails may not be cut on patients with circulation problems, diabetes, and those taking chemotherapy drugs.

> Passive range of motion exercises require a doctor's order. [In most hospitals this is an expected nursing function.]

> A nursing care planning conference is held daily for each team. The conference and patient to be discussed should be planned in advance and noted in the assignment sheet. The result of the conference should be placed on the NCP on the Kardex. [This was typically not followed on the Oncology Unit.]

Nursing Presence at Charles

The nursing office was in the oldest section of the hospital, away from the mainstream of the public areas. A small bulletin board outside the office held a few standard course announcements from area educational institutions, often posted long after they were useful; a poster announcing a program on breast cancer at a nearby university was still hanging a month after its date of presentation had passed. Considering the number of continuing education programs available in the area, there was a dearth of posted announcements. There were no posted weekly or monthly master calendars of staff education at Charles and no articles of professional interest to the nursing community.

The Inservice Education Department office was on the second floor. Next to it was a long bulletin board that was always covered with announcements of continuing education programs for physicians; there were none for nurses. In the main lobby of the hospital, a glass-enclosed case carried announcements of weekly medical staff meetings, conferences, and grand rounds. There was nothing comparable for nursing. In short, there was nothing to indicate lively or active group interest in staff education or involvement with nursing issues at Charles.

When asked her view of staff education programming, the director of Inservice Education responded, "We don't believe in Wednesday afternoon matinees." It was her view that inservice education was best conducted in small groups on each ward. When the researcher commented on this to a nurse, who as a clinical instructor had taught students on several patient units, the nurse said, "Charles is just backing into the twentieth century. What I have seen on these wards called 'patient care' would make your hair stand on end."

Recruitment

Charles usually recruited a high percentage of its nursing-school graduates to become members of the nursing staff. However, because of the fiscal crisis, only five members of the most recent class were hired, and there was such a delay in establishing these five jobs that "the cream of the crop went elsewhere," said one of the faculty. A nurse-recruiter had been employed by the Nursing Department, but when she resigned because of marriage, the position was abolished. The Personnel Department became responsible for recruitment as well as initial screening of job candidates. During a severe staff shortage on the Oncology Unit, the researcher noticed ads in two city newspapers for "RNs, Medical-Surgical, 7-3 with rotation." She asked the unit supervisor, "Why don't they advertise specifically for the Oncology Unit?" Frances replied that Personnel wouldn't use the term "oncology" because the state department of health did not recognize it as a specialty.

Two months and no replacements later, an ad appeared for "RNs Oncology 7-3 with rotation." Up to this point, staff nurse rotation to the evening shift had been minimal, mainly to cover for vacations of the evening staff nurses. But newly hired staff nurses had to agree to rotation in case the needs of the department changed. These ads did not attract full-time staff. The director of nursing explained, "There are seasonal peaks and valleys, and I don't care where you go, any director will tell you the same. February is bad; so is April-May. If they don't admit to this, they're not leveling with you. There's nothing you can do to change it."

Applicants approved by the Personnel Department were interviewed by the director or associate director of nursing, one of whom had to give hiring approval. A supervisor also interviewed the applicant; then the Personnel Department performed the mechanics of the hiring-in process. The head nurse did not interview applicants for positions on the unit. She might accidentally meet such candidates if she happened to be on the unit when the candidate was being escorted on a tour by the director of nursing or the supervisor.

Orientation

A week-long general orientation program for new nursing staff was conducted by the Inservice Education Department once a month or more frequently if there was a large group. There was no difference between the orientation for LPNs and that for RNs from different level programs. When the researcher attended the first three days of a session with three RNs and two LPNs, the whole group was given a packet of information in a folder labeled "RN Orientation." The last two days of the week's program were spent mostly on the clinical unit where the employee would be working. The program involved some didactic material; introduction to some key nursing personnel and their roles, such as the public health coordinator and utilization review nurse; a pharmacology pretest; charting rules; fire films and regulations; personnel policies; and a walking tour of the hospital.

Values, norms, goals, and expectations were part of the presentation. Some comments by the instructor were:

Values. Read the philosophy of nursing when you get time.

Nursing has a lot more say in this hospital since the director of nursing became an assistant hospital administrator.

We do team nursing here, but not all units do it the same, that is, all units are not at the same level. It's a philosophy, and if you try to work it out functionally, it doesn't work.

The team leader is responsible for nursing care, to see that tests get done, the treatments get done. She may not do the actual care, such as washing patients. She is supposed to keep the head nurse in touch with what is going on. The team members report to the team leader. There is the possibility that the team leader is an LPN, though this isn't ideal. But some LPNs do very well. Some RNs would not accept the responsibility of being a team leader when we first started team nursing, but the hospital expects this of RNs. You have to pick up some managerial skills.

You are expected to do your nursing care plans. The joint commission and the state have been very forceful in pulling these nursing care plans. We have a running course for this. [There was no course during the research year, and the supervisor and head nurse didn't know anything about a "running course."] We're doing it according to Mayers. You can borrow a book from the library.

Goals. The goal is for the nurse to be a health teacher here, but we're not there yet. We're not sure how the doctors will accept this, not sure if the nurses see themselves as ready.

The desk work has gotten enormous. We really need a unit manager. That may be our next step.

Norms. The nursing policy book has been under revision for two years. It is the first time nursing has had our own policy book.

There is a pharmacology course here which all LPNs must take.

There are job descriptions for the graduate nurse and the LPN. The LPN does much of what the RN does, but always under the supervision of the RN

Aides can do enemas and irrigate colostomies.

Expectations. There are things that you can teach without having a formalized teaching plan. What somebody needs to know about insulin, digoxin, hypertension—the things they have to watch for—these are things that you can pick up and point out to these patients. [There was no formalized patient education department or program at Charles Hospital.]

A staff-level nurse must work every other weekend. Linen is delivered only on Saturday on the weekend, so you can make Sunday as light a day as possible.

You can take only two weeks vacation at a time. You can have accrued sick time to thirty days (one day a month) and eleven holidays, including two personal days. If you are sick more than three days, you must have a doctor's slip when you return. Read disciplinary action in your handbook.

There is a card available on the unit for each nurse to keep a record of her continuing education programs. The supervisor will look at these cards at evaluation time and consider employees' initiative at keeping up.

The director of nursing stated that she would not "let go" of a sufficient orientation period on the unit. "It's four weeks average before they're on their own." However, after the first week, this orientation was done "on the job," with one exception. Every LPN and RN had to be supervised and "passed" on medication administration by an inservice education instructor.

Nursing Inservice Education

This department consisted of a director, three full-time day instructors, and one part-time instructor for the evening shift. The director of the department, Mrs. Louise Carson, had returned to nursing on weekends at Charles about seven years earlier, after an absence of twelve years. During her absence she had acquired a degree in education (not nursing) and was asked by the previous director of nursing to be the director of inservice education. Louise was studying part-time for a master's degree, but not in nursing because it was "very expensive" and she had children in college. Irene Floof, the instructor who conducted the orientation, had been absent from nursing for nine years and had reentered the field through a job in a nursing home. She had worked in the Charles recovery room for a year before joining the Inservice Education Department. She had had no formal education beyond the hospital diploma. Both Louise and Irene had graduated from hospital schools about twenty-five years earlier, and both had taken a Nursing Process course within the past three years.

Lois and Annette, the other two instructors, came to the department about midway in the research year. Annette had been a staff nurse on the Oncology Unit for about eighteen months after her graduation from a baccalaureate nursing program, and this unit became one of her inservice responsibilities. Lois, a hospital school graduate, joined the department after receiving her baccalaureate degree in nursing from an NLN-accredited university nursing program.

There was clear evidence of strain in the department. Annette and Lois, the junior members, were trying to expand the educational emphasis from procedures and skills and make the department more professionally stimulating and more accountable for teaching patient care concepts, nursing care planning, and professional issues. The only widely publicized educational offerings that the researcher observed during the year were organized and presented in the late spring by Annette and Lois, who stated that they had met with considerable resistance from Louise, and Irene "agrees with everything Louise says." One program, which nurses from all units were invited to attend, included a preview of a filmstrip series on death and dying, which was repeated several times during one week and was well attended. An instructional program on how to do and teach breast self-examination was held in the hospital auditorium and was also well attended.

When the researcher went to the inservice office to keep an appointment with Louise, the three other instructors were there. Since it was a relatively small room with four desks, the researcher suggested going someplace else to avoid interrupting the others' work. Louise said, "No, they're used to interruptions." After awhile the other instructors participated in the discussion. The researcher asked Louise about the department's philosophy, structure, and responsibilities. Louise explained that each instructor was responsible for the inservice education on three medical-surgical units; she, herself, was responsible for one unit and the coordination of the department. In the specialty areas, such as Intensive Care, Obstetrics, and Pediatrics, supervisor-clinicians were responsible for inservice education. Louise published their list of presentations along with hers in a combined monthly report.

The supervisor-clinician from obstetrics came in during the interview, and Louise suggested that she describe what she had done so far that morning. She said:

> I replaced staff who called in sick; took the night report for the departments from the night head nurses who are really supervisors; made patient rounds; closed a short-term surgery unit for the weekend; oriented a new nurse to medicines; wrote payrolls for six departments; checked all plugs on electrical outlets; and checked lids on garbage cans.

When asked why she did the latter two tasks, the instructor replied, "These are housekeeping functions, but nursing checks to see that housekeeping has done its job."

In describing her department, Louise said:

> It is better to teach on the unit to influence patient care rather than through Wednesday afternoon matinees. More people are contacted on small units. Things like tracheostomy care, injections. Reaching small groups is more efficient—there's better feedback. The inservice person should direct the supervision of procedures, not the unit supervisor. A supervisor is a disciplinarian, too. An educator is not a disciplinarian.

Louise was asked if her department oriented nurses to the Standards of Nursing Practice produced by the ANA and endorsed by the state board of nursing. She did not understand what was meant by the question, although these standards were part of the Nursing Process course that she and Irene had taken. Louise responded:

> You mean the Department of Health standards? They make up their own every year. Now they are zeroing in on nursing care plans like the joint commission, but care plans are not in their published standards book. They are in the joint commission's. Inservice does the initial teaching of nursing care plans. They're coming along here.

The director of the Inservice Education Department and the director of nursing were dues-paying but inactive members of the ANA and its state and local districts. None of the inservice instructors, nor the supervisor, head nurse, or registered nurse staff of the Oncology Unit were members of the professional association.

Annette, the newest instructor, stated that she had not been given any orientation to the inservice department, although she had attended a regional "forum" of hospital inservice directors with Louise. "All they did," said Annette, "was knock BSN graduates and the state nurses' association."

Annette and Lois sought out the researcher to tell her that much of what Louise had said about her own role as an instructor on one unit and about the role functions of the instructors was not "our view of reality." The emphasis in the department was really on "doing as little work as possible," they said. For example, Annette and Lois wanted to revise the department's objectives and job descriptions, but Louise would only put a new date on the old ones. Lois lamented, "I've been the sixth nursing instructor in three years at my desk, and I don't know how long I'll last." The researcher inquired about the fate of the others, and Lois replied, "Some went to Special Tests, like Sherry, she's in the cardiac exercise tolerance lab. She was a BSN graduate who was really good in this department. Some go to teach in the school of nursing." Four months later, Annette left the department to teach in the school of nursing.

The researcher asked Louise about the policy for nurses attending continuing education programs sponsored by other agencies. Her reply was:

> Mrs. Bowman allows budget for outside programs, but she diverts anyone with a request to this office. Our department staff's expenses come from our budget, but the others' expenses come from the nursing office budget. Who goes depends on who went to the last one and who the supervisors recommend who will come back and relate information to other people. Mrs. Bowman is Solomon.

Clare Nelson, an evening-shift LPN on the Oncology Unit, enrolled in an area continuing-education one-day offering given by an enterostomal therapist to teach nurses the lastest techniques in caring for patients with ostomies. She went on her own time and paid the $25 registration fee, "because I thought I might benefit in the future when caring for patients like Mr. Jason who had terrible skin problems." At the conference Clare saw three inservice instructors from the hospital and Vivian Nichols, an LPN from the Oncology Unit day shift. Clare expressed surprise to the researcher that another LPN had had all her expenses paid and received her salary also. The researcher suggested that Clare might be reimbursed for her registration fee if she asked the department, but when she asked, she was refused. Vivian had gone only because at the last minute the fourth inservice instructor was unable to go. A staff member from Oncology was selected because many patients on the unit required ostomy care.

When the researcher attended a local conference on breast cancer sponsored by the American Cancer Society, she saw three inservice instructors and one staff member from EH II. She teasingly said to Annette, "What is this? The budget for outside programs goes to members of the department unless they have another obligation?" Annette indicated that this was the way things were. They were the resource people and had to keep up with new developments. But when asked, "What about sharing those new developments with the rest of the

Charles Hospital nurses? Would the department put on an ostomy program for all the nurses?'' Annette just shrugged. There was no ostomy program during the remaining seven months of the research year.

Chapter 3
The Oncology Unit

STRUCTURE

During the "gaining entrance" period, the researcher had not asked to see the Oncology Unit or to have it described, though she wondered what it looked like. Her earlier experiences of the environments in which cancer patients received care had left both good and bad impressions. Was it significant that the building was relatively isolated from the main wings of the hospital? The dirty, dull gray exterior of the old building called to mind an earlier student experience in a major metropolitan area, in a fourteen-bed ward for the indigent poor, many of whom had cancer, and another impression from a prize-winning novel:

> The double doors to the ward were kept wide open, yet as he crossed the threshold Pavel Nikoloyevitch was assailed by a damp, fusty mixture of smells, partly medicinal. With his sensitivity to odors, it was hard to bear.
>
> The beds stood close together. They jutted from the walls, separated only by the width of bed stands, and the aisle down the middle of the room was barely wide enough for two persons.
>
> . . . the patient in the aisle turned to him . . . and said: "Here comes another cancer" [1].

The Oncology Unit was located on the second floor of the building on the northeast corner of the hospital property. This building had been erected fifty years previously for dormitory and classroom use by the school of nursing.

After the nursing school was moved to new quarters in the late sixties, the interior of the old building was gutted and rebuilt. New plumbing and wiring were installed, and air conditioning, an elevator, and furnishings were added. The first two floors of the building were to be for ambulatory, self-care patients. The first floor connected directly with the old parlor and foyer of the original nurses' residence, which was made into a large patient lounge with a dining room and kitchen. Meals were served family style, and self-care patients could help themselves to snacks. The second floor (EH II) was to be for patients who required instruction prior to discharge, such as those with diabetes.

However, the anticipated demand for self-care and teaching beds was never realized. Gradually, as area oncologists began admitting more patients, they wanted a unit where nurses were more knowledgeable about the care of cancer patients than in the general wards of the hospital. Dr. Green, in particular, the nurses recalled, started admitting patients with leukemia to EH II for chemotherapy. Four years prior to the start of the research, when Charles Hospital opened a department of nuclear medicine and radiation therapy, EH II officially became the Oncology Unit, an experimental unit in hospital care of patients with advanced cancer.

This change from the care of relatively well patients to advanced cancer care was significant with regard to the holdover nursing staff, since their motivation for being there was different from that of nursing staff who came later, most of whom had chosen to be assigned there, or at least were aware of the nature of the unit before they accepted assignment to it.

From the west side windows of the Oncology Unit, patients looked out at a row of tenements; directly below on the north side was a newly paved major city artery. At night, the highway street lamps cast a pink glow through the dirt-streaked windows of the four rooms facing north toward the downtown section of the city. At the southeast corner of the second floor, an enclosed bridge connected the Oncology Unit with one of the two newest wings of the hospital, built in 1960. All of the "add-ons" connected in some fashion to the central hundred-year-old original wooden building, which was still in use. The patchwork arrangement of the stages of modernization became evident to Oncology Unit patients who were transported to the Radiation Therapy Department, located in the basement. The Radiation Department itself was attractively decorated with bright walls and carpeting, but access to it was through a narrow, dusty, dark, dungeonlike passageway with exposed overhead pipes.

On the researcher's first day in the field, a sunny May morning, the supervisor and head nurse took her to the unit by the "back way" from the nursing office. They walked through the employees' cafeteria in the oldest section of the hospital. It had a sagging, dull, linoleum floor and long, old-fashioned windows without shades or drapes to relieve their drab appearance. When the laundry machines on the floor below were operating, the tables and chairs vibrated. The month before the start of data collection, the local newspaper had reported that the state health department had ordered the cafeteria closed for several days because of sanitary violations.

The researcher, the head nurse and the supervisor then walked through the first-floor self-care unit to an elevator that took them up to a second-floor stairwell. To the right, a door led to the open-air bridge to the second floor of the original nursing school, now used for office space. This open-air bridge was a source of concern to the nurses, since it was easily accessible by patients through the unit's side door to the elevator and stairwell. The nurses expressed some concern that patients in extreme suffering could fall or jump off the bridge, although no patient ever did. For example, one day, Mr. English, a quiet, reserved patient, had been found disoriented and shouting on the bridge, and in his state of confusion it was not easy to get him back into the building. (That was the beginning for Mr. English of a several-day period of complete disorientation, thought retrospectively to be due to drug reaction to Methadone and electrolyte imbalance.)

As she walked into the unit, the researcher was pleasantly surprised. The sun coming through the doors of the patients' rooms brightened the yellow wallpaper in the corridor. It was quiet, there were no odors, and the ambiance was more modern than that of the older administrative sections of the hospital, thanks to the dropped ceilings and other reconstruction. It was a short distance to the nurses' station.

Ordinarily, patients and visitors came to EH II by the main access routes, either from the parking garage, which was connected to the hospital's rear second-floor entrance, or up one flight from the main lobby. On the second floor of the main building, signs saying ONCOLOGY UNIT pointed the way through a medical-surgical ward of the newest hospital wing. All stretchers and wheelchairs going to and from EH II had to pass through this ward, as did patients, visitors, and hospital personnel. Here the corridors always seemed noisy and congested. In one area, desks used by medical students lined the corridor on both sides. Sometimes patients were tied into chairs outside their rooms. Some of the rooms had three beds in space that seemed designed for two. Opposite the nurses' station of this transit ward, halfway down the hall on the right, a mobile medication cart was almost always in use by a nurse. A red plastic sign on the top of the cart senselessly said "QUIET PLEASE, MEDICATION NURSE."

At the end of this ward, the corridor turned right to the Oncology Unit. A doorway led to a small dark foyer that narrowed to the enclosed bridge to the unit. The original renovation plan called for furnishing the foyer-bridge area as a patient lounge, but this had not been done. A bed with orthopedic attachments and a manikin was stored in the foyer and took up much of the useful space. The bridge had windows about two-thirds of the way down on both sides, so that on a sunny day this area was warm and bright, even though the windows were streaked and dull.

Sometimes a patient would take a chair out there for a change of scenery, and before the unit became really short-staffed, one of the aides, Alice Boardman, would often wheel a patient out there to sit and talk. In the cold weather the bridge wasn't used much because it was unheated.

Across the bridge, to the right upon entering the Oncology Unit, was a small conference room used by the nursing staff for staff meetings or conferences and also by doctors for writing on charts or making business calls. It was furnished with a table and four chairs, a telephone, a narrow bookcase, a file cabinet, and a built-in dresser. This room also had a bathroom and thus was often used as a private room for a patient with an odor problem or disorientation due to delirium tremens (DTs) or other organic brain syndromes. When that happened, the furniture was moved out of the conference room onto the bridge.

Beyond the conference room the floor divided into an "L" shape, with the congested nurses' station in the right angle. As one faced the nurses' station, the right side of the back wall opened onto a tiny open room with purse-sized lockers and coat rack for the staff on one side and two straight chairs on the other. Nurses sometimes sat here to read or write on a patient's record, and the researcher often sat here to record field notes or read charts. Behind this room was a staff lavatory. The head nurse, Karen Foster, and a staff nurse, Annette Brown, shared a locker. On the researcher's first day, after introducing her to staff members at the desk, they gave her the lock combination and told her something that was to be a theme for the entire year. "Be sure you lock it after you use it. We've had a problem with thefts. Two of the nurses have had money taken from their wallets."

Adjoining the nurses' station was a glass-enclosed medicine station with cabinets, a double-locked narcotics box, a refrigerator, and a sink. This station was rarely used, because the newer system for dispensing medicines required using two large carts, which when not in use were kept in the corridor opposite the nurses' station. The carts had a drawer for each patient, and once a day the pharmacy courier would remove the entire drawer and replace it with one that contained the patient's drugs ordered for that twenty-four-hour period. The nurses used the top of the carts to prepare narcotics and other injections, additives for intravenous infusions, and other types of medication. From the point of view of noise, distraction, interruption, and physical displacement, the carts were in the worst place on the unit, but there was no room available for their storage.

Patient rooms were on both sides of the corridor, on both ends of the "L." Each of the seven two-bed rooms and three three-bed rooms had a bathroom with sink and toilet. Each patient had a modern adjustable-height electric bed, a bedside stand, and overbed table, and a small, built-in dresser-closet combination, which provided some storage space for belongings. Near the nurses' station were men's and women's shower and bathtub rooms, though these were hardly ever used, because many patients were too weak and many had radiation markings on their skin that were not supposed to get wet.

Unfortunately, the researcher's pleasant first impressions of the unit's ambiance were not lasting. When the sunshine dimmed, the once-bright yellow walls were seen to be faded to a mustard color. No draperies or curtains decorated the dirt-streaked windows, which were especially noticeable at night, and the window shades were dirty and worn. The traditional white hospital bedspreads didn't do much to liven up the patients' rooms. No paintings or pictures relieved the dullness of the walls, except in one three-bed room where two unframed and frayed travel posters were taped to the wall.

Some patients, however, made the alien space of their hospital room considerably more personalized. Mrs. Dionne taped all her greeting cards to the wall, and by the time her two-and-a-half months of hospitalization were over, most of the wall space was covered. Others put up drawings done by children or grandchildren; some kept small photos of loved ones in sight. Rebecca Lewis, transferred from another hospital for radiation therapy for lung cancer (she was told before transfer that it was the "curable kind"), was cheered by the staff for her interior decorating. She brought with her a Persian-type rug, several large throw rugs (which she also supplied to her roommate), floral-patterned bed linens, and a quilted, floral bedspread. She also wore her own lingerie and stylish loungewear. At forty-one, she was vibrant and alive and as colorful as she made her living quarters. When she was transferred downstairs to the self-care unit, her room looked like a modern motel. Rebecca lived for just four more months.

Rita, a registered nurse who came to the unit from another part of the country in the spring, ten months after the start of the research, had some difficulty adjusting to the unit. She stated, "If I was a patient, I'd just like to lay down and die. Next to the suffering, the surroundings are negative, and the unit is always short of supplies."

While the aesthetics left a lot to be desired, structural deficiencies created more critical problems. Because the rooms were originally constructed as classrooms or residence rooms, the heads of most beds were in alcoves or hidden by walls. It was possible for the staff to see only six patients from the hall, and these only if the door was fully open. Except in these few cases, a nurse could not make a quick check on patients as she walked by a room. She had to walk all the way into the room and turn left or right. Some patients, not wanting their roommates in constant view, kept the curtain pulled across the foot of the bed. While this arrangement afforded some additional privacy, it also meant that some patients were disturbed unnecessarily when they were resting. Also, with no patient lounge, this structural shielding reduced social contact and cut down on serendipitous meetings of patients and visitors and chances for sharing information or building support. It also reduced the staff's opportunities for observation of patients.

Because of the original building construction, modern wall oxygen and suction outlets were not available. There were many patients with respiratory deficits from lung cancer or complicating pneumonia, who required oxygen, which had to be supplied in cylinders kept at the bedside. Mobile suction machines were used when necessary.

When the building had been gutted and refurbished, the steam radiator system had not been replaced, and the heating system on the Oncology Unit was an almost continual source of patient complaints. Even on the coldest winter days, some rooms were stiflingly hot and dry, which made it more difficult for patients to cough up secretions. Other rooms were never warm enough in winter.

The air conditioning was uneven, too. One evening a patient threatened to sign out because it was too cold in her room. The patient, an angry, thirty-eight-year-old woman with lung cancer, had a persistent, nonspecific fever, which her doctor could explain only as a phenomenon of "widely disseminated disease." Annette, the charge nurse, knew that if she adjusted the thremostat, other patients would complain that their rooms were too warm, so she covered the vents with silver duct tape.

The housekeeping was a source of constant complaint. One day, the researcher heard the charge nurse, say to the clerk, "Mae, call housekeeping. The curtains around the bed in 221 are full of old feces. Tell them to wash the floor, too. It's filthy."

Dr. Fisher commented, "The air conditioning is poor. There are no screens—flies come in through the windows if they open them. The housekeeping is poor, the rooms are dirty. One of my patients came in and refused to stay. If you don't believe me, go upstairs and look around EH II [a gynecologic unit]."

The housekeeper, Mabel, was described by the head nurse as "not a good housekeeper, but she's the third one we've had this year. Trying to get this place adequately cleaned is like hitting your head against a brick wall."

One evening the researcher was in the conference room discussing the death of a patient with the chaplain. He interrupted her, saying, "Excuse me, but there's a set of antennae over your left shoulder." It was a huge roach emerging from a bag of food scraps that had been left on a pile of clothes on a chair. The conversation ended as Father Joe sealed the bag and took it out of the room.

Another evening, while talking with Ellen, a graduate nurse, in the conference room, the researcher kept hearing noises in the light fixture on one wall. Finally she said, "Ellen, I hope I'm not hearing things; but aren't there noises coming through that light fixture?"

Ellen calmly replied, "Oh yes, they're the rats behind the wall. The cold weather has probably driven them in from the new construction site. The patients hear them scurrying behind the walls all the time. They complain about the noise."

The head nurse told the researcher that a patient, seeing a mouse in the bathroom, threw up all over the floor. Another mouse was seen by a visitor, who locked herself in one of the patient's bathrooms until she was assured that it had been removed.

During an orientation class, the inservice instructor said the "Johnny Mop" problem had been going on for five years. The maids thought the nurses should change the disinfectant solution in the Johnny Mop jars, and the nurses thought the maids should do this. One year the state health department observers noted that no one was doing it. In the last week of data collection, the head nurse said that the dispute about the Johnny Mop jars was still going on; the Housekeeping Department was supposed to empty them, but didn't. The head nurse said, "I can't stand looking at them."

Since the hospital stay was long and many patients were a long way from home, some of the cluttered look around patients' beds resulted from their personal belongings, as well as from dressings and other equipment. Some of the nursing staff were more fastidious than others about straightening up. One time Mr. Neil, a college chemistry instructor with a pathologic hip fracture corrected by surgery, was attempting to grade student final-exam papers. When he returned to the unit after receiving radiation therapy, he "chewed out" the nursing technician for daring to rearrange his papers—he knew just where everything was.

The staff tried to keep odor to a minimum by paying attention to patients' personal hygiene and by keeping dressings, wounds, and drainage bags clean. On occasion, however, these efforts were not effective. For example, Mr. Frank was transferred from a three-bed room to the conference room after a visitor and one of the staff had vomited from the odor. Mr. Frank had been admitted in a toxic condition; he had an ileostomy that was draining, as well as other drainage sites on his abdomen. He lived for two more days, and the odor permeated the entire unit, most noticeably around the conference room and the nurses' station. On autopsy, Mr. Frank was found to have deep, intra-abdominal abscesses, which accounted for the odor. The head nurse said, "We used every electric deodorizer we had and put deodorizer drops on the sheets and dressings and kept him clean, but nothing worked."

Mrs. Belofsky, who was admitted with gastrointestinal bleeding and diarrhea, was receiving blood transfusions and treatment to stop the bleeding. When Dr. Thomas and the head nurse went to see the patient, the researcher went along with them to the three-bed room. Mrs.

Belofsky, whose bed was in an unventilated alcove, told Karen she wasn't getting off the bedpan until the bleeding stopped because the bloody stool constantly dripped out of her. As the staff left the room after seeing another patient, Mrs. Luckman, she signaled for Karen to come over. Mrs. Luckman whispered that she couldn't stand the odor. Karen told her they would try to take care of the situation. On leaving the room, Dr. Thomas said, "That room stinks."

The odor lessened as Mrs. Belofsky's bloody diarrhea became controlled. Opening windows, using electric deodorizers and deodorizer drops, and prompt emptying of bedpans provided some measure of environmental odor control.

Mrs. Luckman's problem with the room odor was not her major concern. She was an elderly lady with lung cancer, but the primary site was unknown. She had been hospitalized on EH II six weeks earlier for chemotherapy and was discharged without pain. She had been given Adriamycin as an outpatient, but this had to be suspended because her white blood cell count had become depressed. She was readmitted with chest pain in the upper scapular area, difficulty in swallowing, and hoarseness due to left vocal cord paralysis. She had been on morphine for pain relief. The lung cancer had advanced, but radiation oncologists could find no specific lesion to radiate, and because of her low white cell count they did not want to give her nonspecific radiation. She could have gone home except that she could not give herself injections for pain relief, and her daughter worked.

Dr. Thomas said, "Let's see how you do on this oral medication."

"That won't help," said Mrs. Luckman.

The doctor said, "Let's try." Mrs. Luckman retorted, "I have to have needles."

He said, "I can be as stubborn as you are." Mrs. Luckman sat with a pouty expression on her face. "Look," said Dr. Thomas, "you have four options: you can give yourself injections, your daughter can give you injections, you can go to a nursing home, or you can go home on oral medications." He then explained how the first was impossible, the second wouldn't work, the third was not necessary for her level of need, and the fourth was the best solution. Mrs. Luckman was unconvinced.

The doctor said, "Look, let's try. While you're here, if it doesn't work we can always go back to the neddle."

The patient was obviously not happy; she then turned to Karen with her complaint about the odor. Mrs. Luckman did go home on oral medication, but her daughter was also taught to give her mother injections for pain. Since the daughter worked in a shop she owned not far from her home, she was able to return when her mother did not get sufficient relief from the oral drug, give the injection, and return to work.

Nurses' Station

The nurses' station consisted of a stand-up counter that shielded a lower desk from the corridor. The low desk, with its three chairs, was used by nurses or doctors for charting; the patient charts hung on a rack in back of the desk. On the far end of the counter was a stack of notebooks, including a log book of admissions and discharges, a message book for the staff with updates on policies and procedures from the head nurses' meetings, and an attendance book for unit staff meetings and conferences. Visitors to the unit stood at the counter to talk with nurses or the ward clerk, and occasionally they would stand there while recording notes on patients' charts.

All of the patients' charts were kept at the nurses' station; it was rare when at least one was not in use. Behind the long desk, which could accommodate three people comfortably, was a wall with a bulletin board and a closet that contained policy and reference manuals. The space between the desk and wall was just wide enough for one person to pass at a time. The ward clerk occupied one of the chairs and sat at the far end of the desk by one of the two telephones.

The nurses yielded territorial rights to the charting desk to the doctors, who generally pulled all their patients' charts when they came on the unit for rounds. Usually only one doctor was on the unit at a time. Students complained that Dr. Fisher was very possessive of desk space and wouldn't move to let them get past or use the desk. "He could do a quarter turn and be out of the way," one student griped. The nurses' station was the most public place on the unit, because to get to any of the patient rooms, visitors had to pass it. Two patient rooms were directly opposite, to the right of the station, and the patients nearest the doors could certainly hear what went on, some of which must have been disquieting. Staff were not always discreet in their verbal communications. For example, one day Vivian Nicols, an LPN referring to a newly admitted patient, commented loudly to no one in particular, "What is this, another colostomy? What are we running, a colostomy center?" Vivian, who often muttered and mumbled around the medication cart, grumbled one day, "I have seven patients, and every other team has five." (When the researcher looked at the assignment sheet later, she noted that Vivian had the fewest patients of any of the teams, and none of the teams had seven.)

In describing events, the staff sometimes used terms that an outsider would not understand. An RN came out of the conference room one day with her plastic-gloved hands in the air and announced, "Mr. Hoover exploded." The researcher didn't realize what she meant, and everyone else just looked. As she walked by, Terry grimaced and said, "Diarrhea."

On three occasions an aide stopped at the desk about 5:30 A.M. to pick up the night report. Her friendly but loud greeting in the quiet of the night easily could have awakened patients, but none of the staff seemed to mind. When the researcher shuddered, a nurse remarked, "Oh, she's terrific."

The morning (seven o'clock) and late night (eleven o'clock) change-of-shift reports were given at the nurses' station. The afternoon (three o'clock) report was given in the conference room, if it was empty, or in a treatment room.

Two Kardexes, one for each wing, were kept at the low desk. Each patient's Kardex contained essential identifying information and a condensation of his or her care, including medical orders, treatments, observations, and diet as well as a space for nursing orders (the nursing care plan). In Charles Hospital, however, separate medication Kardexes were kept on the medication carts, and no information about the patient's medications appeared on the main Kardex. This was said to be for cost-accounting purposes, since a duplicate copy of the initialed medication Kardex went to the pharmacy as part of the drug charge system. Nurses initialed the medication Kardex to indicate that the patient had received the drug ordered. No record was made on the nurses' notes about routine medications, but nurses were supposed to comment in the notes on patient responses to medications. This was often not done. In order to get a composite picture of the patient's regimen, one had to use both Kardexes. For example, some cancer patients had secondary diagnoses of hypertension or chronic congestive heart failure. These secondary diagnoses were often not written on the main Kardex, but the medication Kardex would show that antihypertensive drugs or digitalis preparations were being given. There was no way to know who was accountable for the observations connected with these drugs—the nurse who gave medications to all patients in her team or the staff person assigned to the patient, who usually used only the main Kardex.

One effect of the "center stage" location of the nurses' station was that there was no private, quiet place for nurses to sit and think. The head nurse had no office, and the conference room was often occupied. Patients, visitors, or other hospital staff who stopped at the high desk were able to overhear staff interactions and one-sided telephone conversations. For example, one time Mrs. Luckman's daughter, Mrs. Carr, was talking at the nurses' station with Angie Williams, the public health coordinator. Mrs. Carr was on the visitors' side of the nurses' station, and Angie was on the opposite side. She had telephoned a supply store to see if Mrs. Carr could stop on the way home to purchase a certain soft restraint for her mother, because it was softer than the restraints used in Charles, and Mrs. Luckman was "skin and bones." Mrs. Carr did not want her mother, who was becoming more confused, to be injured if she attempted to get out of bed without assistance.

While Angie was "holding" for an answer, it was obvious that Mrs. Carr was listening to the coversation at the other end of the desk between the head nurse and the evening-shift nurses about a patient who, the evening before, was supposed to have received an intravenous solution with added medication. The nurse who had been in charge of medications the night before was unreachable by telephone. Karen was asking two others who had worked the evening before if they knew about the medication. The nurses couldn't say definitely whether the patient had received it. Such overheard conversations could easily erode patients' and visitors' confidence in the nursing staff.

FUNCTIONAL ASPECTS

In the early seventies, when the Oncology Unit was being considered, there was no precedent known to the nurses and doctors at Charles for such a unit in a community hospital. Information was obtained by the nursing supervisor and a staff nurse through visits to a specialty cancer hospital and a medical center with a cancer treatment unit. In Dr. Fisher's view, stated during the research year, which was four to five years after the unit was started, "The unit has developed without any major trauma to the hospital, and there is a lot of respect for the unit."

The unit was primarily for medical treatment of patients with advanced cancer, that is, metastatic disease, and for those with complications of the disease or its treatment. Patients initially diagnosed as having cancer while on the unit were the exception. Patients requiring primarily gynecologic or surgical treatment of cancer were admitted to other wards. When a patient on the Oncology Unit required surgery, he was transferred postoperatively to a recovery unit, and when his immediate postsurgical condition stablized, he was returned to EH II.

Two years after the unit opened, a report on its development and progress was published in the county medical society journal. The report was written by Dr. Ben Fisher, chief attending oncologist at Charles and medical director of the Oncology Unit, and three nurses—the supervisor (Frances Kiely), a staff nurse (Mildred Hawes), and a former head nurse. It was stated that the article was written to describe the unit's progress, to explain its problems as well as its advantages, and to emphasize the interdependent relationship between physician and nurses, which was required for the success of such a unit. This statement and the physician-nurse coauthorship seemed, to the researcher, to be a significant departure from traditional nurse-physician relationships at Charles Hospital.

It was impossible for the researcher to assess retrospectively (two years after the publication) whether the article's statements were idealistic or reflected the reality at that time. However, many of the activities described in the article were nonexistent when the researcher was on the unit, and some activities had changed significantly. One item that was not used during the research year was an orange worksheet, which was supposed to be the first chart page. Its purpose was more rapid and efficient communication on nonurgent problems among individuals involved in the care of the patient. Also not used was an active "problem list," to be kept on the inside of the chart cover, which stated both the patient's and the family's concept of the illness. This had been found especially useful by house staff and consultants. The head nurse said regretfully that she had probably discouraged its use when she first came to the unit (one year before the research started) because there were so many other problems of greater priority.

Dr. Fisher did use a problem-oriented method for recording medical progress notes. Once a week he restated the problems, and under the heading "Concept" wrote the patient's perception of his diagnosis and, if different, the family's. He was the only physician to record in this manner. There was no problem-oriented system used by the nurses, either in planning or recording nursing care.

The article mentioned "Weekly nursing conferences" with Dr. Fisher, allowing for "in-depth discussion of general floor problems, specific patients, or for didactic lectures on chemotherapeutic agents or investigational drugs," but these were never held during the research year. A family discussion group was cited in the article as helpful in assisting families to cope with the stresses of the disease and in getting answers to specific questions from representatives of nursing, social service, and chaplain's service as well as peer support from other families. The discussion group was terminated halfway through the research year, after a period of decreasing viability. A plan to have each staff nurse spend a day in Dr. Fisher's office to get a more well-rounded picture of the field of oncology was not active; the invitation was open, but only one part-time member of the current staff had done this, at a time when she was becoming depressed over the many tragic patient situations she observed on the unit.

"Weekly interdisciplinary rounds with representatives of physical and occupational therapy, social service, and nursing, including the public health nurse coordinator" were never held, and in the researcher's view, they were sorely needed. There was interaction between the head nurse or charge nurse and the other individuals involved in a patient's care, but there were no interdisciplinary group conferences about any patient's care.

The article also mentioned a patient questionnaire concerning their care and any suggestions, which was to be completed and returned after the patient was discharged from the unit, but this questionnaire had been discontinued not long after its inception. When asked the reason, the supervisor replied, "Because the hospital wouldn't supply the stamps." Initially, patients were asked to return the questionnaires before they left the unit, but this raised questions about the validity of the answers, since the patients were still captive. About thirty had been returned. Basically, the questionnaire was a check-off list, with questions such as, "Was the staff courteous?" to which the patients checked "always," "usually," or "never." One suggestion for improvement was "Better temperature control—either too hot or too cold and no humidity." General comments included, "Nurses more friendly; rooms not so dingy"; and "My wife and I were in this unit as patients and cannot say enough for Oncology Unit EH II. Thank you." In response to the question "Is the floor quiet at night to allow you to rest and sleep?" there was one poignant response, "Patients cry at night."

A factor that may have limited the success of the original proposals for the unit was that the head nurse, who had been there for a year before the start of the study, was the fourth head nurse in the four and a half years since the unit had started. Relocation and marriage were the reasons given for the resignations of the previous head nurses.

Another probable limiting factor for some of the discrepancies was Dr. Fisher's time. When the article was written, Dr. Fisher was in partnership with Dr. Green, but two years later, that partnership broke up. Dr. Fisher began a solo practice primarily in oncology, while Dr. Green went into hematology practice and only rarely admitted a leukemia patient to the Oncology Unit. He said, "I don't admit there any more. It's personal, and I don't wish to divulge the reasons." The head nurse stated that Dr. Green told her in an apologetic way that his failure to admit patients to the unit had nothing to do with her or the nursing care.

When the researcher spoke with Dr. Fisher about three months after the field work started, he stated, "I'm not as idealistic about the concept of an oncology unit now. I'm not sure that the oncology unit is workable in a community hospital. Patients don't get enough support."

"You mean emotional support?" asked the researcher.

Yes, things are said in front of patients which shouldn't be said, like, "It's so good to see somebody walking out of here." I'm sorry we're losing Annette. She's a college graduate. We should keep four-year college graduates on this unit. The nurses should have continuing education. We [doctors] should help but don't. I'm really screening patients now. I wouldn't admit a twenty-seven-year-old with Hodgkin's disease to this basic environment. [He did admit young patients with other malignant diagnoses who required intravenous drug protocol.] You've got me when I'm down. The floor has a weak supervisor. It's her responsibility to look after the nurses. I've withdrawn my interest in the unit. Look, I have to be in the office by twelve o'clock. But I will talk to you. How long will you be here doing your study?

Another possible factor in the unit's failure to reach its original goals was the supervisor's perception of her role.

> I'd really like to function as a clinical supervisor, but you can't in this hospital, anyway. They really need a clinical supervisor full time. If you go in a room and a patient wants to talk to you for whatever reason, you want to stay; but my time is divided among three different types of units. The trend toward administrative supervision has gotten stronger in the past three years. There's a lot of personnel work—getting involved with people's time off, leaves of absence, committees.

SPECIALTY UNIT CHARACTERISTICS

One way to assess a subculture is to examine how its cultural characteristics differ from those of the larger institution. According to the article in the county medical journal, one of the staff's goals was to convince the nursing administration that the Oncology Unit was a specialty unit like Coronary Care and Intensive Care, whose needs should be examined independently of other units. There were several ways in which this difference was established. In hiring, if there was a vacancy on the Oncology Unit, a nurse would be told about the type of unit it was. The director of nursing stated that when she spoke with potential staff about oncology nursing she gave a positive view, stressing problems as well as rewards, but a number of prospective staff said they didn't want any part of it.

Another way in which the unit's specialty nature was acknowledged was through the biweekly rap sessions for nursing staff conducted by Ted Craffey, the head nurse of the Psychiatric Unit. These sessions were primarily for the well-being of nursing staff rather than for resolution of patient care problems. It was thought that if the staff resolved some of their interpersonal difficulties, they would be a more cohesive group, better able to deal with the inherent stresses of the work.

Another indication of the unit's special nature was its support group specifically for families. Also, the chaplain, Father Joe, visited all the patients daily, as he did in the Intensive Care Unit; he visited patients on other units a few times a week unless they requested otherwise. He also served as a friend and supporter of the nurses and was a member of the family conference team.

Admissions and Transfers

A special system existed for admitting patients to the Oncology Unit and for transferring them within the unit. Instead of going through the admissions office, the doctors gave to the head nurse or charge nurse the names of new patients to be admitted from home or another facility, and these were listed in chronologic order in a book kept at the nurses' station. When a bed became available, the first patient listed was called in. Charge nurses said Dr. Fisher had a way of helping to decide whether certain patients shouldn't come to the unit. "He says, 'Do you have a nice room?' meaning do you have a roommate or room situation that will be nice for my patient." The charge nurse would then review the vacancies with him.

If a patient had to be admitted in an emergency and no beds were available, he or she was admitted to one of the regular units of the hospital and then transferred to the Oncology Unit if a bed became available and no one was on the waiting list. The only exception to this was that patients who were to receive hepatic artery infusion therapy were given priority, since they required specialized nursing care.

Under this system nurses had the right to move patients around on the ward for greater roommate compatibility or convenience of observation. For example, Mr. Cirri in a two-bed room was moved to Mr. Tallini's room, because both were first-generation Italian-Americans who, it was anticipated, would have common interests. Barry, a thirty-five-year-old man, who was dying "by inches," as Dr. Fisher wrote, was moved directly across from the nurses' station for closer observation. Mrs. Varney, hospitalized for several weeks in a three-bed room, had had two roommates die. When a dying trajectory was predicted for another of her roommates, she was moved to a two-bed room with an ambulatory patient. On the other hand, some patients did not want to be moved, such as Mrs. Kaye, who had been through a death experience with one roommate but chose to remain with another obviously dying roommate.

There were times when the nurses would have liked to move patients but were unable to do so. For example, if a large majority of the patients were men, little could be done to move a woman patient since the rooms were unisex. An exception to this rule was made for a married couple, the Streets. She was admitted for radiation therapy for cancer of the kidney, and he, for cancer of the gastrointestinal tract, which required colostomy surgery.

When Mrs. Street was asked, "How do you feel about your room arrangement?" she replied, "It has its advantages and disadvantages. I worry and get involved and don't get my rest sometimes." The researcher asked if the Streets had requested this arrangement. "No, the doctor [Dr. Long] did, and my husband and I went along with it."

Time was an important factor in compatibility moves. In the beginning of the research year when the unit was most fully staffed, such moves were made frequently, but after the departure of two full-time staff nurses, and a heavier workload because of the admission of sicker patients, elective moves became a low priority.

Standing Orders

After much discussion, the head nurse and supervisor were able to convince Dr. Fisher and Dr. Long that the patients would benefit if certain standing orders could be initiated by the nurses. The nurses were concerned with such problems as having blood available and starting transfusions early in the day while the IV team was on duty, rather than having an inexperienced intern trying to do a venipuncture in the evening and the patient receiving blood late into the night. No house staff (interns and residents) were assigned to the Oncology Unit, and the attending doctors were not always readily available by telephone. For example, Dr. Fisher did consultations in hospitals as far as forty-five miles away; Dr. Long had two offices, admitted patients to two hospitals, and maintained a research laboratory in a medical center in a nearby state after he went into solo practice. On certain weekends it was sometimes several hours before he returned a call to EH II.

The standing orders that were developed to deal with this problem were, "Type and cross match and hold two units of packed cells for hemoglobin below 8.5 and hematocrit below 27"; and "For excessive bleeding start a 'keep open' IV of 500 cc NSS." In a revised version, other orders included medication for constipation and diarrhea and moist or excoriated skin associated with radiation therapy. A standard mouthwash solution prepared by the pharmacy (½ teaspoon salt, ½ teaspoon sodium bicarbonate and one pint water) was to be used by all patients unless otherwise ordered, because of the potential for mouth lesions from treatment.

It was important, however, for the doctors who admitted patients to the unit to agree on one set of standing orders so a meeting of the three oncologists, the supervisor, and the head nurse was scheduled. Dr. Terwilliger, one of the radiation oncologists, was asked to attend as a consultant, and the researcher was invited by the nurses. Dr. Long brought along an intern who was doing special studies for him, but Dr. Fisher dismissed the intern from the group, stating he was not a member of the staff of EH II. With some adjustments, the orders were approved and signed by Dr. Fisher and Dr. Long. The latter's associate at the time, Dr. Thomas, did not attend and refused to sign orders because he said he wasn't specifically invited to the meeting. Later, after he went into private practice, he signed an expanded version of the standing orders, although he specified that he wanted to be called immediately if there was any change in one of his patient's condition. Since the standing orders were only for the Oncology Unit, they did not have to be approved by the Executive Committee of the medical staff. Dr. Terwilliger suggested that a conference group be formed to share discussion of interesting cases, but the group was not formed.

Critical List

In other areas of the hospital, patients in risk of death were put on a "critical list." Since the researcher noted no official observance of this on EH II, she asked the head nurse about it. Karen stated, "The doctors keep the families well informed, and if there is a sudden change in condition, we call the family."

This happened in the case of Mrs. Juan, who was forty-seven years old and was known to the staff from previous admissions. This time, she was hospitalized for many weeks with widespread gastrointestinal cancer. She was ready to be discharged several times, but complications, such as septicemia and pneumonia, intervened. She became increasingly weaker, had pain, and was markedly cachectic. About three o'clock one afternoon, Mrs. Juan vomited blood. The head nurse tried to get the doctor and also called her family, who lived quite a distance away. An evening-shift graduate nurse, Ellen, stayed with Mrs. Juan. When Dr. Long phoned in and was told about the hematemesis, he debated whether to put in a nasogastric tube and attach it to suction to remove the blood. He called a gastroenterologist who had treated Mrs. Juan previously. Ellen said:

> I'm glad he ordered the n-g tube, otherwise she would have continued to vomit the blood. She didn't seem to realize that she was dying until she started to bleed. She kept saying, "I'm going to bleed to death." We kept saying, "No, you're not." She said to her four sons, "Please make up before I die." She started to get confused. One of her sons and I stayed with her. Dr. Long arrived at ten o'clock just as she took her last breath. He pronounced her dead. I hate to get attached to my patients but I got attached to her. I feel bad. The gastroenterologist said she had such a beautiful brain and her body is just wasted. She was literally exsanguinated.

Ellen, a twenty-one-year-old hospital school graduate, left the unit after seven months when she failed her state licensing exam for the second time.

MILIEU

During the day, particularly from eight in the morning until noon, there was a sense of busyness on the unit, with many patients going to and from other departments on stretchers and in wheelchairs, as well as food trucks, supply carts, and personnel going to and from the unit. The traffic was particularly heavy on Mondays, when the treatment departments and diagnostic laboratories resumed operations after the weekend. Any patients admitted over the weekend were scheduled for special tests and X-rays on that day, and the frenzy of activity frequently caused the head nurse to say, "I hate Mondays."

Although a sign on the side door to the unit said "Visiting Hours 1 to 8 P.M.," and the official hospital policy was, "No children under age 14," visitors, including young children, were allowed to come at any hour of the day or night if they discussed the situation with the head nurse, who was very flexible in this regard. A few times, doctors wrote orders concerning visitors on the order sheet such as, "Family may stay all night" or "Five-year-old son may visit." Ambulatory patients were generally permitted to have visitors in the lounge area of the Self-Care Unit on the floor below, and parents with very young children usually brought them there.

A daytime-pass policy enabled patients with their doctor's permission to leave the hospital during the day on weekends and holidays and be back by seven or eight at night. For example, Mr. Laird, a businessman with brain metastasis from prostate cancer was receiving radiation therapy, but since the department was closed on weekends, he was permitted home on a pass with his tax accountant so that he could get his income tax prepared on time. His wife was at home with advanced cancer and could not come to the hospital, so it afforded a visiting opportunity also.

Many patients expressed regret that there was no lounge or solarium where they could sit and talk. Some did form small groups and gather at the north end of the floor where more wall space was available. There was a small kitchen on the unit, but it was open only to staff. Clare, an LPN on the evening shift, was very concerned about patients' nutrition and stated:

> Patients should have their own kitchen instead of routine house diets. They should be able to get a poached egg or something palatable when they feel better after their chemo. Last Saturday everybody on house diets got hot dogs and sauerkraut. Sure, they don't have to eat what's on the tray, but then they lose out on their nutrition and they need that. The cook should be orientated to oncology patients.

Boredom seemed a common problem, with relatively few patients providing their own diversions. Some read books; Mr. Lampe made placemats on nailed frames; Mr. Crosson did jigsaw puzzles continuously; Mrs. Knull did crossword puzzles. Small televisions could be rented, but on the whole, the researcher was impressed (or depressed) at the amount of time that patients spent lying in bed with no diversion at all. Some nursing students commented:

> That place is very stagnant.

> There's nothing for the patients to look at. Can you look at TV all day? Out the window? Yuk.

> I'm not surprised that some of those patients go off the deep end. Mr. Graves back there. All he has to do is look straight ahead at a curtain. They

ask what it's like outside. They want to know the news. There's no calendars. All they know is it's some time during the day.

On the other hand, Janet was a nursing student who had cancer of the ovary (it was removed, but she had subsequent lung metastasis), and she was admitted periodically for chemotherapy. She told her classmates, "Sometimes you don't want to talk to anybody. You feel so sick you want to be alone."

One of the aides, Jill, noted that the whole unit seemed more cheerful one cold January day because during the night there had ben a four-inch accumulation of snow. The patients in rooms facing the streets with a view of the snow were in better spirits and were eager to hear what it was like outside. Jill felt that boredom was a problem for many of the patients, and the snowfall gave them something new to think and talk about. Boredom was especially noticeable in evenings when the ward quieted down after the hustle and bustle of the daytime activities was over. One of the evening LPNs became pregnant early in the research year. Her delivery date became a topic of conversation among some of the patients, who verbally "counted down" the days before her due date. Three of the patients had performed this same activity when her first baby had been expected two years previously. Patients also cautioned her to avoid excessive physical stress in her care activities.

The "float" ward clerk said, "You can tell this unit is different because of the expressions of the visitors' faces. On the other units they're more relaxed, some are even jovial. Here they're somber."

Work Pace

In most hospital areas, there are seasonal variations in the patient census because of reduced elective admissions during holidays, medical meetings, or physicians' vacations. On EH II, however, there were no such slow periods. During most of the research year, the physicians were in solo practice and did not take extended vacations. Occasionally, different internists would provide weekend coverage for Dr. Fisher and Dr. Long. When Dr. Fisher took a one-week vacation in January, he arranged for an internist to cover for him with backup by an oncologist in a nearby state. He said, "It's taken so much to plan for all the eventualities that I wonder if it's worth getting away."

This sustained work pace caused considerable dissatisfaction in the nursing staff around the Christmas holidays, since with staff taking time off, the workload was actually increased. At one conference, an aide said, "You promised me a letdown [of the pace of work], but I've been here five months and it hasn't slowed at all." The only time the unit slowed down was in the spring when one room at a time was closed for painting.

At three different times during the year, four patients died within a few days, which was particularly stressful for the staff. Though the beds were quickly filled with new patients, comments such as, "I feel as if a burden has been lifted," were not uncommon. Staff acknowledged that they were all affected by a bad mood or a down period of one of the nurses or doctors or a "run" of very sick patients.

PATIENTS' ATTITUDES

In the article published by Dr. Fisher and the nurses, it was stated that the quality of care on EH II must have been apparent to the patients, since the majority wanted to return to the unit when they had to be read-mitted. Apparently the trauma of hospitalization was lessened by knowing that they would be cared for by nurses with whom they were familiar. But a small minority of patients did not wish to return to the unit because it was a "cancer floor." While some patients could state their feelings clearly, it was recognized in the article that others might be equally uncomfortable but not able to verbalize it. It was thought that the problem for some patients was not the unit itself, but the fact that ambulatory patients became depressed about critically ill or dying room-mates. The article stated that no patient was admitted if they did not wish to be there.

One day the researcher made rounds to the regular hospital wards with Dr. Fisher and the nurse from his office. One lady started crying and complaining bitterly about the lack of attention. Dr. Fisher said to her, "I told you about the special unit you could go to where the care is better, but you tell me you don't want to go there." She was discharged shortly after that, but on her next admission she consented to be admitted to the Oncology Unit.

Numerous comments indicated that patients felt that EH II was more acceptable than the rest of the hospital. Mr. Wells, a seventy-eight-year-old man with lung cancer, who was receiving radiation therapy, was so upset with his care on another unit that his family asked Dr. Fisher to transfer him. A lovable gentleman, Mr. Wells could only shake his head, almost in horror, when asked about his transfer. "I'm happy to be here after being on that other floor. My nephew is happy, too." A few months later, a "thank you" card from Mr. Wells' family said, "Although he has passed away, we are sure he was as grateful to you as we are."

Most of Dr. Fisher's patients knew that it was a cancer floor, unless the family did not want the patient to know his or her diagnosis. Dr. Fisher said 98 percent of his patients knew their diagnosis; 2 percent did not. The 2 percent included very young children; very elderly patients with no particular family connections and no interest in knowing, who only wanted to know it was a tumor; those who had a need to deny and trust the doctor; and those whose family insisted that the patient not be told—"This sometimes involves a battle with the family," said Dr. Fisher, "but the family wins out." Rarely, relatives did not want the patient to know the diagnosis of cancer, and this wish was respected by the doctors. "It is mainly for support that this occurs. Families believe they can better support the patient."

However, this did not mean that patients lacked perception. Vivian, one of the LPNs, said one day a patient asked her for a medical dictionary and looked up the word "oncology."

When he came to the unit on a stretcher, Mr. Breen, who had been bedridden at home with advanced lung cancer and now had pneumonia, observed the direction sign that said ONCOLOGY UNIT. After a few days, as he recovered slightly from the pneumonia, which had left him very sick and weak, he asked Lisa, one of the staff nurses, "What does oncology mean?" She told him it meant "diseases of cell division." She sensed that he wanted to know the truth, but she knew the family didn't want the diagnosis told to him. Lisa went to the head nurse for help and asked that the family be advised of the patient's questions. Dr. Fisher wanted him to know also. At a family conference attended by Mr. Breen's wife and sister, the wife said, "I told Dr. Fisher . . . well, you're the doctor, but I'm his wife, and I know him better. He would just give up if he knew, because his sister died of that." Mr. Breen died a few days later.

Dr. Long acknowledged that there was "probably less depression" at Overhill Hospital, where his cancer patients were mixed in with others on the general wards. He also said:

> Some patients don't want to come back here, although that is not as frequent since the care has improved since Dr. Foster came. In the other parts of Charles, care of the cancer patient is fragmented. Nurses want to ship them over here as quickly as possible. Nurses get depressed over cancer patients because of experiences in their own life.

> Some patients don't mind coming back here. Once they accept that the disease is cancer, then they don't mind coming back here because they get better care. If they accept the disease, then they accept a cancer specialty unit. From the doctors' point of view, care is better on a specialty unit.

Dr. Thomas said "yes and no" to the concept of an oncology unit; "yes, because there's better nursing care; no, because it's tremendously depressing for some patients." His first preference was to admit cancer patients to EH I (Self-Care), then to the Oncology Unit. "The rest of the hospital has abominable care," he added.

Some of Dr. Long's patients were not told they were going to be admitted to a cancer floor. One evening the researcher introduced herself to Marge Holland, who said, "Oh, you've come to watch me crawl the walls. Well, my doctor didn't tell me I would be admitted to a cancer unit."

"How do you feel about it?" the researcher asked.

She answered, "I looked around and I asked myself . . . is this what I'm going to be like in three or six months?" When asked if she had adjusted to it, Marge replied, "I don't like it, but I can tolerate it. I just want to get out of here. I want to go home to my own bed." She kept the curtain drawn between the two beds in the hospital room because she found her roommate's argumentative behavior offensive. Marge was forty-seven and had liver metastasis after a malignant melanoma had been removed a year and a half earlier. She died less than a month after this conversation.

Mrs. Parmelli was admitted for radiation therapy to her lower leg for metastasis from breast cancer. After being in the hospital for three weeks, she was due to go home the next day. The researcher asked her about her stay at Charles. Mrs. Parmelli turned thumbs down, but was careful not to proceed until she was again assured that her comments would be confidential. She then replied, "This is my first time at Charles, though I've been hospitalized three times at Overhill Hospital for the cancer. I know what I've got but I don't like to be faced with it from everybody else. At Overhill Hospital, they mix the patients up."

The researcher responded, "You mean you don't like the idea that cancer patients are grouped together on one unit?"

I don't like it at all. You see too much that's upsetting, and you wonder if that's going to happen to you; and I have enough to just deal with myself. There are other things, too. At Overhill Hospital there are showers in the bathrooms in the patients' rooms. Here I have to go down the hall, and of course, with my leg like this I can't trust myself to go that far safely, though I did walk to the bridge just to get out of the room the other day. I try to wait for this bathroom. I do wait as long as I can, and I do understand that patients are in there doing their irrigations and things, but it's inconvenient. And I'm not used to male nurses doing things for female patients. Last night during the middle of the night a male nurse came in to give one of the ladies a bedpan. If I knew in advance, I would never let that happen to me. You asked me how I felt, and I'm telling you.

The patient was asked what had helped her get through this difficult time. She replied:

Well, my husband comes in every day. He is so good. He's been with me all the way. My doctor says I'm a living miracle. I've had cancer since 1971. They never did remove my breast, you know. They just cleaned out the tumor, and then it recurred, first in the nodes, now a hot spot in the leg. I've been on chemotherapy since 1971, and now the R.T.

In contrast, Mrs. De Lilla had been on other units in the hospital and on EH II several times. She commented, "I like EH II, and I don't mind that we're all cancer patients. No matter how bad I am I see somebody worse."

STAFF ATTITUDES

The oncologists continually stressed to nurses and patients that cancer is a chronic disease, with the same principles of treatment as other chronic diseases. Dr. Fisher compared the chronicity of cancer with that of other diseases in which there are periods of exacerbation and of remission, such as multiple sclerosis, emphysema, and arthritis. But the doctors acknowledged that this view is not widely accepted.

Dr. Long said, "A lot of doctors don't even want to treat cancer patients. Once they hear the diagnosis, the patient's dead as far as they're concerned."

The head nurse said that ordinarily, a patient being admitted to the Self-Care Unit was escorted from the Admissions Office on the second floor of the main building through EH II and then down by elevator. But some doctors told the escort not to take their patients that way. They had to go up to the third floor, cross the bridge at that level, and take the elevator from three to one. "How can you expect the public to deal with cancer when some of the professionals can't?" the head nurse asked.

Although no interns or residents were assigned to the Oncology Unit, house staff were called during the evening or night for emergencies or to start or restart transfusions and infusions. Since they rotated assignments monthly, they were not well known to the staff, but many of them asked, "How can you work on a unit like this where everybody's going to die?"

The Charles nursing school instructor commented that students didn't want to come to the unit, because they had learned by word of mouth from other students about the chronicity and downhill course of the disease.

Karen, the head nurse, explained her feelings about this:

> I worked in ICU before I came here. The doctors and nurses ask, "How can you stand working on oncology after working in ICU? Isn't it depressing?" I really don't think it's as depressing as ICU, having patients on respirators for weeks who you know are not going to make it to any meaningful life, or having young men in accidents who die before the night is over. Here I'm able to provide some nursing care, pain relief, and caring, sharing in the people's last months of their lives. I get satisfaction from that. I don't get depressed about deaths. For some of these patients, it's a relief when death occurs, that their pain and suffering is over.

Interestingly, the three members of the nursing staff who had worked on EH II before it became a cancer unit had negative views. Mildred, an

RN, said, "It's a tragic mistake to have all cancer patients together. I thought nurses should rotate. It's successful as an experiment, but I would not recommend it."

Vivian, an LPN, said, "I don't think they should have a terminally ill floor."

"Is that what you think this floor is?" asked the researcher.

Vivian answered:

It is, it is. That's the way I feel about it. I do see a lot of patients go into remission. It appears that when a patient with cancer on the other floors gets real sick he comes here. I don't want to think of cancer that way because my sister has cancer; she's only thirty-three and has been in remission for two and one-half years. Now I think of it as a chroniclike thing. I've changed my view, but not from my experience here—from a personal experience. Oh, my God, if I have to get an illness, don't let it be cancer.

But Janet, the senior nursing student who was undergoing chemotherapy, said, "Many are relieved to get here because they're shunned and whispered about on the other units. 'She has cancer' . . . and nobody wants to go near them. They feel good here; they're not all alone."

Later, speaking to her classmates at a group interview, Janet said:

Cancer patients want to be treated like human beings. They want to talk and to laugh. A patient said to me, "You're not afraid of me are you?" I said, "No" She said, "Even my family won't talk to me." I told her that her family was probably scared and that's why they don't talk. She has a sense of being abandoned. I know how she feels. When I was diagnosed and had my surgery, I wanted to talk so bad, and everybody shut me off.

Janet also described another conversation with a patient who was depressed about losing her hair as a side effect of chemotherapy. The patient told Janet, "You couldn't possibly understand what I'm going through; you're young and you have your whole life ahead of you."

Janet said, "Then I told her again that I could understand, and I took off my wig so she could see for herself."

COMMUNICATION PROCESSES

Several modes of communication between patients and staff were significant, in addition to face-to-face interaction and patients' records. If a patient needed something from the staff, he or she pushed a button on the call bell, which activated a light above the door and at the nurses' station. However, the lights were not always answered promptly, unless the aides were at the desk. Patients sometimes used other methods of calling; it was not unusual to hear a favored member of the staff called for by her first name—this could be an aide, a practical nurse, or a registered nurse. An angry or confused patient might call by throwing a urinal or other piece of equipment on the floor. This happened more often during the evening or night hours.

One afternoon about four o'clock, the call light over the door of room 220, which was closest to the medication cart, was flashing. Sara, a relief RN, was pouring the six-o'clock medications and didn't respond to the light. Finally, the newly admitted patient shouted out from her room, "I have a lot of pain, and I need something for it."

Sara answered from the hall, "You'll have to talk to your doctor about that when he comes in."

"When will that be?" the patient asked.

"I don't know. You were given something at three o'clock, and you only have an order for every four hours." Although the overtness of this incident was uncommon, it illustrates a recurrent problem of pain assessment and management, particularly on the evening and night shifts.

There were two telephones at the nurses' station and one in the conference room. The ward clerk was supposed to answer the telephone, and in her absence any nurse at the desk answered. Patients also had bedside telephones, which were used mostly to receive outside calls. Occasionally, a patient would call a relative or the doctor and complain about his care. Mrs. Green, a patient's wife, told the researcher that she called Dr. Fisher's office two days in a row because when she came in in the late afternoon to visit Barry, his IV had run out.

One afternoon, when the head nurse was conducting a staff conference, the clerk called her to the telephone. When Karen returned, her face was red. She quickly adjourned the conference, saying that Dr. Fisher had called him to say that Mrs. Wiley was "in agony" because she needed an enema. Ruth, an LPN in her first year of practice, said, "But I was with her almost all day, and she didn't say a word. I'll be glad to give her an enema." (The researcher had been in Mrs. Wiley's room at lunch time, and she was complaining of distress then. Ruth was at her bedside also. This was not the only time that Ruth's judgment was questioned.)

The bulletin board behind the nurses' station held the time sheet, administrative memos, announcements about inservice classes or staff conferences, and thank-you cards and notes from patients and families. Near the bulletin board, clipboards hanging from hooks held daily lists of patients' diets and temperatures. A concrete post at the end of the desk often had notices taped on it such as:

Call Rightway (Aide Training Program) instructor for post-mortem care.

Call Dr. Fisher at his home from 6 P.M. to 10 P.M. rather than answering service. After 10 P.M. please call house physician first; and if important, let house physician call Dr. Fisher.

The chalkboard in the conference room was blank most of the time, except for a recurring list of suggestions for spending a sum of money given to the unit by the relative of a patient who had died after a long stay. (Initial suggestions from the staff included the purchase of plants, a coffee pot, a rocking chair. and furniture for the bridge. Eight months later it was decided to purchase some nursing textbooks and a small radio for the unit.)

A public-address system was used to page doctors, supervisors, or instructors; the sound was much more noticeable during the night.

OTHER DEPARTMENTS

The head nurse or the charge nurse spent a considerable amount of time relating to other departments to coordinate patient care and keep the unit running smoothly. For example, they had to schedule diagnostic tests and treatments in other departments; communicate with medical consultants; discuss situations with other nurses who had single role-specific functions, such as utilization review, infection control, or intravenous therapy; obtain supplies; and organize getting patients to other departments on time. "Troubleshooting" was also part of the head nurse's role. For example, if the Radiation Therapy Department was behind schedule and a patient from the unit was delayed there, a nurse from EH II might have to take his pain medication or additional intravenous fluid down to the department.

Radiation Therapy

Charles Hospital had two linear accelerators. Usually sixty to seventy patients a day (two-thirds of whom were out-patients) were treated, but during one week in February, ninety patients a day were treated. The length of a course of treatment depended on whether the goal was curative or palliative, as well as on the site of the disease.

A department member said:

> Lung cancer patients might receive 4,500 rads in a period of four and one-half to five weeks. Most metastatic disease requires 3,000 rads over ten treatments. A curative dose for bladder or pituitary cancer might be 6,500 to 7,000 rads in six to seven weeks.

> There are three radiation oncologists in the department, and patients are seen by one of these once a week while undergoing treatment.

Patients often complained that they had to wait too long in Radiation Therapy, especially the ones on stretchers. There was no set schedule, since patients from outside the hospital didn't always arrive on time. If one of the two machines broke down, there were long delays.

The transporters who took patients to Radiation Therapy were strong, young men. At one time, twenty of the twenty-three patients on the unit were receiving therapy. Since many of the patients were in severe pain and almost all were prone to pathologic fractures, gentleness in handling and lifting them was of the utmost importance. But some of the nursing staff stated that the attendants who were slow and gentle got yelled at for being slow, and the ones who were fast and rough got rewarded. They thought some were very rough. One nurse described this situation:

Mrs. Edwards said in the Radiation Department that her foot hurt. They wanted her to get out of her wheelchair onto the table, and her leg snapped. When she was brought back to the ward they told her to get in bed. When June went in to check her after the attendants returned her to bed, she found that the hip was out of the socket. Mrs. Edwards had a pathologic fracture, which required a surgical fixation.

Some of the transporters who came to the Oncology Unit expected a patient to stop whatever he was doing and get on the stretcher. A nursing student described such a situation:

At 8:00 A.M. Mr. Cirri wanted to get freshened up; at 8:02 he started washing; at 8:04 his breakfast tray came. At 8:06 the transporter came to take him to Radiation. Mr. Cirri said if he was able he'd get freshened up at 6:30 A.M., but at 6:30 the night people all run and hide until it's time for them to leave. Then all the day staff come on and listen to the report. Today, I ran down at 7:20 and got him washed; he was grateful all day.

Also there were not enough vehicles. One special stretcher, which allowed patients to be rolled on rather than lifted on, was used for EH II, and there was one for the other hospital departments, but this was not enough.

One young black man, Pete, was singled out by the patients for being gentle and pleasant. It was not uncommon to see Pete managing a stretcher and one or two wheelchairs and cheerfully talking to the patients while moving along. One day Mrs. Lawrence and her daughter asked the researcher how they could get in touch with Pete's boss to commend him. Mrs. Lawrence was being treated with radiation for a pathologic fracture of the lower spine and on her previous admission had had radiation for lung cancer.

Another patient, Mrs. Dionne, was discharged after two and a half months of radiation therapy and treatment of many complications. She left this note:

To Mrs. Foster and all nursing staff on all shifts in this unit (and Pete)—It is impossible to leave here without expressing my deepest gratitude, not just for the care I received in this unit, but for the concern and consideration extended to me. There is more than good nursing service here. There is a lot of "tender, loving care." Nothing is ever too much trouble for the staff to do and they make you feel like "one of the family." To a great crew—thank you so much for everything.

Sincerely, Denise Dionne

One day the researcher saw Pete in the hall looking dejected. He told the researcher he had hurt his back in an automobile accident two weeks before and had been out for a few days. His department manager had called him in the office and said, "I know you're dragging your ass. Now get out there and move it." Pete tried to explain that his back was still sore. The manager retorted, "I don't want to hear any explanations." Shortly thereafter, when there was a vacancy in another department, Pete bid on the job and got it.

Physical, Occupational, and Respiratory Therapy

Many patients received therapies to overcome neuromuscular deficits caused by tumor involvement or to help regain function after surgical correction of pathologic fractures. What went on in these sessions and how the patient was progressing was usually communicated informally by patients to their doctor or to interested nursing staff rather than through any systematic interdepartmental communications such as a daily departmental activity note on the patient's chart.

Mrs. De Lilla was well known to the staff, having been hospitalized several times previously. She was admitted this time for evaluation of increasing pain in her left thigh and loss of mobility. One afternoon she tried to get up from a commode and felt "electric shock" through her leg. She had so much pain she asked not to be moved. "Just knock me out," she begged and was given medication. The nurses had a terrible time getting her into bed. She had sustained a pathologic fracture of the hip and was operated on the next day for total hip replacement. While on the table, the doctors noted that her right hip was fractured also. Her husband had to be called in to sign consent for prosthetic replacement of this hip also. Mrs. De Lilla was taken to an orthopedic unit postoperatively but was eventually transferred back to EH II. She received physical therapy daily and eventually was able to walk with an aluminum walker. She refused to go to wheelchair kitchen training in Ocupational Therapy, saying that she would be able to get around her kitchen herself. Mrs. De Lilla did have periods of depression, but with support and resumption of some mobility, she was well enough to return home.

Some cancer patients went to Occupational Therapy for treatment of neurologic deficits and basic skill training. Once the head nurse asked the department to come to the unit and provide some diversional occupational therapy for sixteen-year-old Susan Graham. They helped her with some paintings on felt and a leather purse. Susan had been transferred from another hospital after surgery for a brain tumor that was not completely removed. After her postoperative recovery period, she started six weeks of radiation treatments. Her roommates were two elderly, sick ladies. When Susan gained some strength, she went down to the lounge on the first floor to watch television or play cards. She also received a pass to attend her high-school graduation. Eventually she was transferred to the Self-Care Unit.

Charles Hospital also had a Respiratory Therapy Department. Technicians from the department frequently came to EH II to give breathing treatments or chest physiotherapy to patients with potential or actual lower-respiratory-tract infections.

X-Ray

Several times the researcher was asked by visitors if she "followed up" on X-Ray, because patients complained about being pushed, poked, and rushed. The researcher told the head nurse or charge nurse about the complaints, but they did not have much influence on the situation.

One morning Dr. Fisher and the researcher were at the desk when Mr. Vandeveer went by in a wheelchair pushed by an attendant. He asked if Dr. Fisher would be there when he got back. "Not likely," said Dr. Fisher.

Mr. Vandeveer stuttered and stammered. "Well, then, I want to discuss something with you. Well, whenever I have to pass my urine, I have to strain hard and then only a little bit comes out, then I have to push again and only a little bit comes out."

"How long has this been going on?" asked Dr. Fisher.

"A few days. Is that tumor growing?" His eyes widened with anxiety.

The doctor said, "Unlikely, but let's take a look." Dr. Fisher asked the attendent to bring Mr. Vandeveer back to bed.

The attendant wheeled him back, and in a disgruntled voice said, "Do you mind if I sit here in the hall?" and to the aide, "They always do this to me."

During his bone scan, Mr. Popiel had involuntary urination. Prior to this incident, urinary incontinence had been a problem for him at night but not during the day. He was very upset and embarrassed; he was also angry. He said:

> Other departments have a responsibility to treat people humanely. All I know is, they said "he screwed up his whole test." I was in pain, had no breakfast and no lunch, and I was cold on that hard table. They told me, "You're not trying to help." I told them, "You're killing me." They said, "Well do you want to get better or not?" They are unprepared people. They are hired just to give them a job. You know what I mean?

Mr. Popiel explained that at a yard sale about eight months previously he had bent down to pick up a record and had felt excruciating pain down his leg. He managed to leave and had three nights and days of excruciating pain before he went to see a doctor. "They cost so much. They rob you," he said. He was in Valley Hospital's Northern and Eastern divisions and then Charles. He commented:

Charles is OK. I'd come back if I had to except down to that X-ray. I told the doctor when I came in that if he could get rid of 50 percent of my pain, I'd be a thankful man. And the pain is gone with that radiation therapy. I started getting radiation as an outpatient, but I couldn't walk. Now I have this pain in my lower foot [foot was grossly swollen]—but the swelling has been there for eight months. If he can get rid of 50 percent of that pain, I'd be happy. Then I'm going to live it up. I'm sixty-eight. This thing here [a colostomy] was a successful operation. I just had to learn to operate it [irrigate it] once a day. Never gave me any trouble. Then the leg. Now this—[pointing to his bladder area]. Always something.

During the research year, Charles Hospital did not have a CAT-scanner (computerized axial tomography), the most modern computerized brain X-ray system. To have this, patients had to be transported to a medical center in a nearby state. If a relative was not available to go with the patient, one of the staff would go. Alice Boardman, the aide, said:

I took Mrs. Henry [a fifty-year-old woman with multiple metastatic sites from breast cancer, including the brain] to Eastchester for her EMI scan. She took it terrible. There was a mix-up in communications. They didn't have an ambulance when we got downstairs with the wheelchair. They decided to take her in the hospital car. She sat in the front seat. She was so sick. We had to park two and a half blocks from the hospital. We waited two hours for an ambulance coming back.

A few days later, after Mrs. Henry died, Alice asked, "Why did they send her for the EMI scan? A couple of days and they're gone. I wonder sometimes if they don't do it to help the doctor—build up a practice, I mean—it isn't going to help the patient."

One afternoon, an elderly, partially deaf man, Mr. Chamberlain, came down to a family conference. His eighty-year-old wife had been admitted the day before and was disoriented and semicomatose. She was admitted with a diagnosis of "brain metastasis or cerebral arteriosclerosis" and was scheduled to go to Eastchester Medical Center for a brain scan. The gentleman said to the group, "Why do more? Hasn't she had enough?" On questioning him, the staff learned that the doctor had not talked to him about further diagnostic tests. The nursing supervisor said she could help him get in touch with the doctor. Later the social worker talked to him on the unit. A few days later Mr. Chamberlain came into the unit carrying a container of ice cream for his wife, who had died while he was on his way to the hospital. The brain scan had been cancelled after he had spoken with Dr. Fisher, whose philosophy was to let patients and families make decisions about their care after he had presented all the facts to them.

Supplies

Supplies came from different departments but were not always available. One day sixteen-year-old Ginny Coleman, who had had chest surgery at another hospital and was found to have lymphoma, needed to have the bottle attached to her chest drainage tube changed. The unit was told that bottles for the drainage unit were not available, not even for cardiac surgery patients.

On other occasions the pharmacy ran out of Methadone ampules, which Mrs. Dunaway needed every two hours. Another time the pharmacy called to say it had no more of the pain medication being used in a research project. They wanted the head nurse to call Dr. Long to get some more, which she did.

One day Lisa asked at the afternoon report if Ellen was coming on. When the answer was no, Lisa said, "I wanted to tell her that she gave Mrs. Mead 5 mg of Drug H instead of 0.5 mg. I don't know what to do about it."

Someone said, "Make out an incident report."

"Well it was the pharmacy's fault and they acknowledged it." There was lots of bowing and curtsying from Annette, a day RN, and Sara, an evening RN, at pharmacy's unexpected acceptance of responsibility.

"How did you find out?" Lisa was asked.

"I called the pharmacy when the med nurse found 5 mg in her drawer."

"How is the patient?"

"She had a good night's sleep. She needed that." A note about the error was posted at the nurses' station for Ellen.

Vicki, an RN, was the team leader for three heavy, weak ladies in 221 who required a Hoyer lift (a mechanical device) to get them out of bed into chairs. She had to borrow one from the Intensive Care Unit. Considering the number of heavy, weak patients who had to be lifted or assisted to stretchers or chairs by the nursing staff, there was a lack of supportive devices readily available. Although the males of a subculture generally do the heavy muscular work, the reverse is true in the hospital subculture. There were no male aides assigned to EH II, and no doctor was ever observed physically assisting a patient. They did call such needs to the nurses' attention.

The researcher noted that after the morning report and before making rounds to patients, the head nurse always went into the treatment room and counted supplies. When the researcher asked her about this, Karen said, "I do count the supplies every morning. I'm not supposed to have to, it's CSR's job [Central Supply Room], but I can't depend on them. I can't take a chance on the staff's not having enough supplies." Sometimes basic equipment such as urinals and bedpans were not available when aides were readying rooms for patients who were on their way to the unit.

Social Service

Mary Hein, the social worker, mainly handled nursing home referrals and family crisis situations. She was a member of the family conference group.

In hospitals today doctors are under pressure by federal Medicare regulations to discharge patients as soon as medically warranted. Patients' charts are reviewed carefully, since any prolongation of a patient's stay must be approved by a Utilization Review Committee.

Mr. O'Toole, an eighty-two-year-old man with bony metastasis from cancer of the prostate, had gone to his local hospital because of increasing back pain. When spinal involvement was found, he was transferred to Charles for radiation therapy. A large-boned, heavy man, he lived with his grandniece, Peggy, her husband, and their four preteen and teenaged sons. Peggy, his nearest surviving relative, was very thin and looked chronically fatigued. Since she was employed part time as the assistant manager of a supermarket, she could visit only two or three times a week.

The question of Mr. O'Toole's care after the conclusion of his radiation therapy came up early in his hospitalization, since he had had a good response to therapy. His pain was considerably relieved and his mobility had increased, but his grandniece had conflict about taking "Daddy Tim" home. After other hospitalizations he had been quite content to retire to bed and have Peggy wait on him. He was very heavy to lift, and as bed rest increasingly lessened his muscle strength, he frequently fell when he got up to go to the bathroom. Sometimes he was unable to get himself off the commode, and she had to call in outside help. A nursing home was recommended, but the thought was intolerable to Daddy Tim. Peggy tearfully expressed her guilt feelings about this on several occasions, but decided it would have to be. "He makes me feel so full of guilt, but what else can I do? I just can't manage him any longer at home."

Peggy was referred to the social worker, who gave her a list of recommended local nursing homes to visit and helped her arrange for Daddy Tim to receive Medicare benefits. Though there were vacancies in area nursing homes, there were no Medicare beds. Nursing homes allot a certain quota of their beds to Medicare patients, and when this quota is filled, they won't take any more, since the Medicare reimbursement rate doesn't meet their costs.

Daddy Tim did not want to use his pension money to pay for the nursing home, so he agreed to go on a Medicare waiting list. However, the Utilization Review Committee said he had to leave the hospital, since his treatment was successful and he was medically able to be discharged. Through the social worker's intervention, he was then transferred to a nursing home as a partial pay patient, that is, he agreed to pay the difference between the home's rate and the Medicare reimbursement rate.

Security

Members of the security staff were contacted on several occasions to schedule transportation for patients going for diagnostic studies at other locations, to report suspicious-looking strangers hanging around EH II or adjacent areas, and to report theft complaints of patients, families, and nursing staff. On a follow-up visit to EH II the researcher stopped at the hospital entrance for a temporary identification badge. The guard asked her if there was anything new on EH II.

"Should there be?" she inquired. He replied that there had been four thefts in two days, including $80.00 from a patient's wallet. This long series of thefts was finally resolved the following month when marked money was placed in the bedside drawer in a room in which both patients were semicomatose. A member of the staff was identified and subsequently dismissed.

Public Health Nursing

Angie Kerr, a registered nurse, worked with visiting nurse associations and homemaker service agencies to arrange for skilled nursing care or homemaker services for patients who were discharged home. She also contacted agencies such as the American Cancer Society, which provided some equipment and funds for certain drugs or services, if the patient needed financial assistance. Angie said:

My job is to provide the continuity of care from hospital to home. Doctors on the Oncology Unit would rather see patients go home than to a nursing home. There are times when families would be more relieved if the doctor said, "nursing home." It would relieve their guilt if the doctor ordered it. Family conferences help. If they hear other families vent their guilt or fear of failure, it may help some families say, "We can do it, too."

She gave an example:

Warren Armstrong had one daughter nearby and one in a distant state. The close daughter had guilt that she could in no way put him in a nursing home. But I had the feeling she couldn't cope. She was sickly. We asked her to come to family conference to listen. We had her check out nursing homes, but she said she would try to care for him at home. I ordered the equipment from a supply house and arranged for the visiting nurse and a home health aide for four hours a day. I came in on Friday, but the doctor decided to hold him until Monday. I came in Tuesday. The daughter had not come in since the previous Thursday. I called her, and she was sick. I feel the impact of that equipment made her ill. They kept her father here for one and a half weeks. Then she came in and finally said, "I don't think I can take him home. Put him on a list for a nursing home." Before placement, he died.

Angie said that Dr. Fisher liked his patients to die at home. For example, she arranged discharge for a twenty-seven-year-old woman with three small children, because Dr. Fisher wanted the family to have every minute together. Her husband wanted her home, and his mother, who was a nurse, could take care of her. She lived for two days after discharge.

Since Angie saw cancer patients throughout the hospital, the researcher asked her if she thought grouping patients on the Oncology Unit was a good idea. She replied, "From what I've seen on that floor, yes. I find a different attitude there."

"What's the difference?" asked the researcher.

Angie replied, "Some kind of a warm feeling. I hate to say this . . . more of a caring feeling than on the other units. They're quick to call me when a patient needs help. I don't find out from the other floors until they're out the door."

REFERENCES

1. Solzhenitsyn, A. *The Cancer Ward*. New York: Dial Press, 1968, Dell Edition, 1974, p. 9.

Chapter 4
The Doctors

OVERVIEW

This chapter concerns the doctors as individuals and their relationships to the nursing and hospital staffs, patients, families, and each other. Significant issues associated with the medical treatment of cancer patients that arose during the researcher year are addressed. Much of the data were gathered by participant observation and informal interviews. Scheduling appointments for formal interviews with the three physicians took persistent effort and wasn't successful for six to ten months. The reasons given were the same for all—too busy and too time-pressured.

The primary admitting physicians were Dr. Fisher, Dr. Thomas, and Dr. Long, all in their late thirties. Dr. Fisher was the medical director of the unit; he was in solo practice and was a board-certified oncologist-hematologist, as was Dr. Thomas. At the start of the research year, Dr. Thomas was associated in practice with Dr. Long, who was not board-certified in any specialty but who had a practice exclusively in oncology, with offices in two communities. In addition to an M.D., Dr. Long also had a Ph.D. in pharmacology.

A short article in the Charles newsletter stated that Dr. Long operated a clinical pharmacology unit at a nearby university medical center and that he was involved there in clinical drug research, postdoctorate clinical training, and medical and graduate student training. Though Dr. Long admitted only cancer patients to EH II, during the summer he did admit a group of medical students to the Self-Care Unit for a week-long study of hypertension drugs. The nursing supervisor, who coordinated the admission of the students, commented, "He makes a lot of money doing research for the drug company, but it involves a tremendous amount of work for the pharmacy."

Dr. Fisher had reviewed and approved the researcher's proposal at the request of the Charles administration, but she did not meet him until the start of data collection. The head nurse introduced the researcher to Dr. Fisher, who gave her a cordial welcome and offered his cooperation. When the head nurse introduced the researcher to Dr. Thomas, he commented:

> Oh, this is the nurse we were talking about over coffee. You're going to write down that I have curly hair, that after two days of good behavior I start bitching? I guess I have to be on my best behavior for a year while you're here. Why did you choose this nursing home for your doctoral study?

The researcher explained the purpose and the methodology of the study. She did not meet Dr. Long until several days later.

The researcher asked each physician how he came to choose oncology as a specialty. Their answers were brief. Dr. Fisher said, "I trained in hematology and oncology." Dr. Thomas answered similarly, "During training in hematology my teachers were also into oncology." Dr. Long said he "just evolved into it."

ROUNDS

At the start of the research year, Dr. Fisher made medical rounds to his patients daily, and Drs. Long and Thomas alternated daily rounds and weekend coverage to their group of patients. Rounds provided an opportunity to observe each doctor's style and treatment philosophy, and the nature of doctor-nurse and doctor-patient relationships. When one of the doctors came in to see patients, he usually pulled the charts for one wing from the rack, put them on a cart, and went from room to room. During the day, the head nurse usually accompanied the doctors on rounds, carrying the drug Kardex so that medications received by patients could be readily ascertained. The team leader might join the group for the patients on her team, but this was not an expectation.

On the researcher's first day, she joined Dr. Thomas; the supervisor, Frances Kiely; and the head nurse, Karen Foster, on rounds. The first of many memorable patients was a thin, dark-haired, fiftyish-looking lady, Mrs. Wanda Wagner. "Who are you?" she asked the doctor.

He explained that he had seen her the day before at Overhill Hospital, "where you were out in left field." Mrs. Wagner's major concern at the moment was that she could not walk. Dr. Thomas pulled the covers off the foot of the bed to examine her legs. Her right foot was rotated outward and looked flaccid; she could lift both legs off the bed, the left moderately, the right only slightly. She asked if she would be able to walk.

He replied, "You need radiation to your head so you can walk again." There was no explanation of the connection between her head and legs, nor was any attempt made to explain what was happening to her. Mrs.

Wagner asked how long she would be in the hospital. Dr. Thomas answered, "At least three weeks." The patient looked upset and stated that her own doctor (the referring physician from her home town) had told her that she would be hospitalized at Charles for two weeks. Dr. Thomas sternly said, "No, three weeks."

Mrs. Wagner stared at the group, looking annoyed at the jocular behavior and the side conversations taking place at her bedside, though she did not verbalize her displeasure. As the group left the room, Dr. Thomas told the nurses, "You may have trouble with that lady. I see depression building." He added that she had been "rammy" when he had seen her the day before at Overhill Hospital. A nurse commented that according to her chart, Mrs. Wagner had a psychiatric history. The doctor said he thought that was probably a mistake.

According to the chart, Wanda Wagner, who was forty-four, was from a small town about forty miles south of Lafayette. Her husband was unemployed, and they had a seventeen-year-old son and a fifteen-year-old daughter. She had had cancer of the left breast and a radical mastectomy two years and two months prior to this admission, her third different hospital admission in less than a month. She had been admitted first to her local hospital with nausea, vomiting, and dehydration. Diagnostic tests "turned up normal." A psychiatric consultation there described:

> a very complicated picture of a depressed woman with conversion features. At time of breast surgery there appeared to be a strong defense via isolation of affect with subsequent reaction formation vis-à-vis involvement with the American Cancer Society. Impression: Depressive neurosis; consider the possibility of a hysterical illness, conversion type or possibly even a psychotic depression.

The consultant recommended antidepressant medication as well as "individual therapy with aggressive milieu support to her. If she is unresponsive, ECT [electroconvulsive or shock therapy] will be considered." The physical examination showed a "weakened-looking female" with "no current physical diagnosis." The recommended nursing approach was:

> Consider self-care.
> Must be in groups.
> No time alone in room.
> Must get self to meals, walking or in wheelchair.

There were unexplained chronologic gaps in the record, but the chart revealed that after two and a half weeks, Mrs. Wagner was transferred to Overhill Hospital for psychiatric care with a diagnosis of "depressive neurosis." There a physical examination showed that she had ptosis of the left eyelid and anisocoria (unequal size of the pupils), and a brain scan showed mutiple areas of metastasis. Her right leg had become so weak that she was unable to walk. When she was transferred to Charles Hospital after a five-day stay at Overhill, Mrs. Wagner was complaining of severe headaches and, in addition to the ptosis and anisocoria, she had bilateral papilledema (swelling of the optic disk due to increased intra-cranial pressure). Mrs. Wagner was admitted to Charles primarily for "palliative radiation therapy to entire cerebral contents, 3,000 rads in two weeks through parallel opposed fields." In addition to radiation therapy, Mrs. Wagner also received triple combination chemotherapy. During the last week of her hospitalization, Mrs. Wagner had her ovaries removed.

With treatment and supportive nursing care, Mrs. Wagner's mind cleared and she was able to walk prior to going home. A few days after her discharge, Dr. Long, who was at the nurses' station talking about some of the unit's environmental problems, disclosed that several of Mrs. Wagner's nightgowns, as well as her breast prosthesis, had been stolen while she was a patient on EH II. "That sort of thing is getting out of hand," he said.

One year later, as the researcher was completing data collection, Mrs. Wagner was readmitted for further radiation therapy to new metastatic sites in her spine. She said that for the most part she had been able to carry on her homemaking responsibilities. Her family was well prepared to help when she needed them, and she took great pride in talking about the accomplishments of her teenagers.

On the researcher's second visit to the Oncology Unit, the head nurse was off and Mildred Hayes, an RN, was in charge. "It's so quiet today," she said; "the calm before the storm. Then Dr. Long will come in and the place will get wild."

The researcher hadn't met Dr. Long at that point, but recalled a comment made about him when she had first joined Dr. Thomas and the nurses on rounds. Dr. Thomas asked Mr. Duncan, who was sitting on the side of his bed receiving oxygen, if he felt well enough to go home; the man's eyes widened over the top of the oxygen mask. After examining his chest, Dr. Thomas told the group that the fluid in Mr. Duncan's lungs was "still halfway up; what drug is he on?" A nurse handed over the Kardex with the list of medications, and Dr. Thomas asked, "Why was Drug X discontinued?"

"I don't know," said the head nurse. "Dr. Long discontinued it and put him on Drug Y."

Dr. Thomas replied, "Drug Y won't work for this, he needs Drug X."

One of the nurses said in an audible whisper, "Dr. Long must own stock in the company that sells Drug Y." After checking through the chart, however, Dr. Thomas found an explanatory statement that Mr. Duncan was resistant to Drug X.

Earlier, when the researcher was completing her arrangements for field study, she heard a comment that was a clue that there were some problems in staff relationships with Dr. Long. One of the staff said, "Now we'll see how research-oriented Dr. Long really is."

When the researcher saw a tall, heavily built, dark-haired man pull several charts out of the rack one morning, she knew that this was Dr. Long. After introducing herself, she explained her purpose for being on the unit. No one had told Dr. Long about the study. "That's soft research; it's not publishable," was his first comment. The researcher responded that some qualitative studies of this type had been published and had been well received.

When the researcher explained that interviewing the physicians was part of the study and that she would eventually like to make some appointments with him, Dr. Long asked, "Are you going to pay the doctors?" The researcher stated that she hadn't planned to, explaining that her research was unfunded, but that she would make office appointments if necessary.

"You could have gotten a grant," said Dr. Long.

"I guess I didn't approach the right group," was the researcher's reply.

Dr. Long continued, "Are you going to talk to patients?" When the researcher replied in the affirmative, Dr. Long said, "Who cleared this, Mrs. Kiely?" (the nursing supervisor).

"Yes," replied the researcher, "and Dr. Fisher, Mr. Smith, and Mrs. Bowman."

Dr. Long then commented, "I was only kidding about the project. Do you plan to share it with the nurses?" When the researcher explained that she couldn't review findings while the project was ongoing, Dr. Long asked, "Isn't there something you can share right now? You must have a bibliography on the readings you've done this far."

With that, a young, curly-haired woman passed by in a wheelchair on her way to X-Ray. Dr. Long gave her a casual greeting. Later, the researcher found from the chart that the patient, Susan Weber, was twenty-seven, married, with two children, ages three and five. The physical exam showed that she had an "atrophic right upper extremity with a functionless right hand." Her chart also revealed that two years and two months earlier, Susan had sought medical care for pain in the subscapular area. She was treated with intra-articular cortisone, and as the pain progressed she was given an orthopedic evaluation and placed in traction. In six months the function in Susan's right hand was gone. Subsequently, cervical adenopathy was noted, but a biopsy of the nodes showed up nonmalignant. During the next year her pain increased, and the function in her hand and arm worsened. About six months before she was referred to Dr. Long, a biopsy of the nodes showed some malignant cells. Dr. Long's admitting impression was: "Sarcoma vs. carcinoma right supraclavicular area with Horner's syndrome.'' Susan was admitted to Charles Hospital for further diagnostic tests, including bone-marrow aspiration and biopsy, and for chemotherapy treatment.

While reading Susan's chart the following day, the researcher was intrigued by a brief nurse's note of the previous afternoon: "Patient upset by diagnosis." Frances, the supervisor, explained that the reports of a biopsy and bone-marrow test had come back after the researcher had left the unit. Dr. Long had gone to see Susan without telling the nurses or taking along someone who could remain with her. He apparently told Susan that she had extensive metastasis but that she would be treated with chemotherapy.

Frances said, "The shock state lasted while Dr. Long was in the room. Shortly afterward, Susan became nearly hysterical and asked the nurses to call her husband." Since their home was a considerable distance away and the husband was at work, it was several hours before he could get to see his wife.

Annette was on the evening shift. When the researcher asked her what had happened, she shuddered and held her head in her hands, saying, "It was awful. I had her husband in here [the conference room] crying for half an hour." Annette said no one was present when Dr. Long told Susan that he "was going to lay the cards on the table—she had the tumor all over." Lungs and abdominal lymph node involvement had shown up on the tests. Annette thought it was terrible to tell Susan like that. "At least Long could have told her with her husband present or told him first," Annette said. She added, with a skeptical look, Dr. Long had told Mr. Weber there was an 80-percent response rate to chemotherapy and a 35-percent cure rate for sarcoma.

Rounds with Dr. Fisher were not problematic in terms of his relationships with patients. As one of the LPNs said, "Dr. Fisher is warm; he sits on the bed, holds the patient's hand, looks right at her, and uses the word 'cancer.' He explains things."

Although the number of admitting physicians was relatively small for a twenty-three-bed unit in a hospital the size of Charles, it was evident that the nursing staff had to relate to three markedly different personalities. Dr. Thomas was more formal with patients compared to Dr. Long, who was more casual in his bedside manner. Dr. Thomas had more of a peer relationship with the registered nurses than did the other physicians. One nurse contrasted the associates, Drs. Thomas and Long, by saying, "Thomas is frank."

The researcher asked, "Brutually frank?"

"No," the nurse replied, "he just doesn't give false hope. Dr. Long gives unending hope."

Another's view was, "Dr. Fisher . . . he's so good with his bedside manner. He'll say, 'there's just so much we can do, and now let's keep him comfortable.' Dr. Thomas is like that. But Dr. Long is not—that's what's frustrating.''

There was a marked difference in the way Dr. Thomas and Dr. Long communicated with patients about their prognoses, Dr. Thomas being more factual and specific. For example, Mrs. Harris, an attractive fifty-year-old with bone and brain metastasis from breast cancer, had double vision, ataxia, and severely bronzed skin and baldness from chemotherapy. Three nurses went with Dr. Thomas to Mrs. Harris' bedside. He asked her how she was, and she replied, "Not good." She had vomited the day before and had pain. The doctor asked if she had received any of the ordered drugs for the pain, and she said she didn't think so. Dr. Thomas scolded her somewhat, saying, "It's up to you to ask if you need something." The medicine Kardex was checked and it showed that Mrs. Harris had had medicine for nausea only, once at 7:00 P.M. and again at 5:00 A.M.

Dr. Thomas asked Mrs. Harris how she did after the intraspinal administration of a chemotherapeutic drug. Mrs. Harris said she didn't notice anything different and asked the doctor what she was supposed to notice. The doctor replied he didn't think one injection would make any difference at all, that she would need several, and it might be three weeks before she would notice any change. He stressed, "If, any. There's no guarantee." He then said:

> Last night we were talking about your situation, and I want to propose this to you. There is a way to get that medication into you without the inconvenience of repeated spinal punctures. They use it for children with leukemia, and it might work for you. Now I want you to think about this. It involves putting a catheter or tube through the top of your skull into the cerebrospinal fluid. There would be a button at the exit of your skull, and the medication would be injected through it; you could inject the medication through it.

Mrs. Harris asked, "I would do it?"

Dr. Thomas said, "No, we would do the injection."

She said, "Who is we?"

"Us, the doctors," was the reply.

Mrs. Harris propped herself up in bed on one arm and said, "Well, I think when it involves something unusual like that, you should talk it over with my husband."

Dr. Thomas said, "All right, there's no rush to this. I want you to think it over." Mrs. Harris, however, deteriorated rapidly and did not receive this special mode of treatment.

Mrs. Kaiser was recovering after a decompressive laminectomy for spinal metastasis, a period of disorientation and a subsequent period of extreme pain. On November 1, she was sitting in a chair when Dr. Long came into her room. As he approached, Mrs. Kaiser started to cry, and the following dialogue ensued:

"Come on Mary. Bite on a bullet. Are you homesick?"

"I'm crying about my son."

"He's at college now, isn't he?"

"Yes, that's where he's supposed to be. He came home for the weekend."

"He came home to see you, didn't he?"

"Yes."

"Well, we'll have to get you better. He'll be home for another weekend."

"No, it costs $186. He can't afford it."

"Well, he'll be home for Christmas?"

"Yes."

"We'll have to get you better and get you home for Christmas."

Contrary to the nurses' expectations, Mrs. Kaiser was eventually discharged, though she was very sick and required a great deal of care.

In his casual and nontraditional style, Dr. Long made some interesting comments about patients. To one family he stated, "She's been going downhill for a year, but she's a tough old bird." He introduced the researcher to a seventy-four-year-old woman by saying, "This is South State's answer to the dirty old man." When told that a patient had voided "600 cc after having voided 3 cc 400 times a day," he commended the patient by saying, "Your wife said she knew you were a great pisser, but she didn't know how great!"

In general, rounds were doctor dominated rather than interdisciplinary. Frequently, the researcher had heard the nurses mention significant information about the patient in a change-of-shift report, but instead of bringing up these matters at rounds, the nurses remained silent, waiting for the doctor to speak. Nurses often seemed casual rather than systematic about reporting to doctors what they knew about patients. Sometimes Dr. Fisher would invite their participation by saying, "Any nursing things?"

Rounds were sometimes embarrassing for the researcher. For example, Dr. Thomas and Mildred would engage in joking behavior in the hall and in a casual, off-handed manner would continue their conversation when they were standing in front of a patient. Though this did not seem to be intentional, one could understand how patients could view such behavior as depersonalizing. On one occasion, the group on rounds with Dr. Long arrived at Mr. Autry's bedside. On the bed was the morning paper with a front-page article on a controversial subject. Annette and Dr. Long debated the issue for several minutes while the patient just looked. Addressing the patient was almost an afterthought.

The group crossed the hall to Mrs. Parmelli's room. She was being treated for bone metastasis in her left lower leg, but had also had a nonmalignant growth removed from her eyelid. The eye dressing had been taken off that morning, and both eyes were blackened. Dr. Long laughed at Mrs. Parmelli's appearance, and Annette said that was how she herself looked after her nose job. Dr. Long looked at Annette's nose, and they discussed having her nose job redone. When Dr. Long turned his attention back to Mrs. Parmelli, he noted a cross that had been marked over her knee to show where the radiation was to be directed. He made a comment about her knee being blessed, and her look of annoyance prompted Dr. Long to remark, "Mrs. Parmelli is not in a laughing mood today—the surgeon just took off the bandages."

Sometimes the nurses did speak up on rounds to learn some essential information. When the group left Mrs. Parmelli's bedside, they went to see Mr. Saul, who had upper spinal metastasis. There were two sandbags near his head. Dr. Long said to the head nurse, "The patient's head is supposed to be between the sandbags; his head shouldn't be resting on one." With an annoyed expression and tone, the head nurse told Dr. Long that she understood that and had earlier positioned the bags properly, but the patient had insisted on putting his head on top of one. Mr. Saul was confused.

The head nurse asked Dr. Long how the patient should be moved, since his chest sounded congested. The doctor did not answer the question directly but stated, "It is a problem because a subluxation of the vertebrae could result in transection of the chord." Mr. Saul then complained of pain. He apparently had had no medication since 2:00 P.M. the previous day. When Dr. Long asked him why he hadn't asked for medication, the patient indicated that he didn't know how to obtain it.

"Just ask one of the girls," the doctor said, "they'll give you something." He turned to go to the next patient. The head nurse persisted. Again she asked how the patient should be moved. "He should be moved like he's on a spit," the doctor said loudly, gesturing with his hands.

The nurse said, "You mean log-rolling?" Dr. Long nodded his head affirmatively.

A clerk came into the room and told Dr. Long that he was wanted on the telephone; he left. Lisa, a staff RN, came into the room and, not seeing Dr. Long, asked, "Where is God?"

"God's on the telephone," replied another nurse.

Nurses sometimes disagreed with a doctor's orders and resented carrying them out, but usually they verbalized this only among themselves. Occasionally, however, they would assert themselves. The staff was annoyed at Dr. Long's insistence that they get certain obtunded patients out of bed. "Get him up," he'd say.

Once Lisa retorted, "You get him up," but he didn't. None of the doctors was ever observed to physically assist a patient, even when the patient looked extremely uncomfortable. Some patients were very heavy, in addition to being very ill and hardly able to sit up. The nurses thought it wasn't safe to sit such patients in chairs, fearing they could slip to the floor if left alone, and staff rarely had time to just sit with a patient.

Some of the team leaders did not participate in rounds. An LPN, Vivian, expressed a negative view:

> I don't think rounds with the doctor is a good idea. Patients have questions to ask the doctor, but they won't do it if a lot of people are standing around. If it was one team leader, OK, but all of them like to go, and some go all the time. This is their [patients'] time, and it really is a short period of time; and they don't get the chance to ask the questions that are really on their minds. You can go behind them after the doctor leaves, and they have a thousand questions; and I say, "Did you ask the doctor?" and they say, "No, I didn't." I wonder if doctors like nurses on rounds for the reason that patients' questions are discouraged.

At a conference, a Charles nursing student asked: "Why do they ignore the patient while talking in the room? You're talking about a person like a person wasn't even there. It's always been that way, and it goes on everywhere, especially on the teaching floors."

Jill, an aide who worked on the unit for about six weeks, commented to the researcher: "I get in on the worries of patients and their complaints. The doctor gets there, and they blank out; a lot of them are scared of doctors—especially the women. I try to get the patients to write out a list." Jill thought the nursing staff could be more sensitive to the patients' needs, "like sitting down with them and asking them what their problems are and helping them make a list. The doctors like the list." She added that the patients who couldn't remember well were the ones who needed the list the most.

Interns and Residents

Rarely, a noncancer patient would be admitted to EH II until a bed became available elsewhere in the hospital. The medical resident or intern working with the patient's physician would see the patient on a regular basis. Also, the intern on call for the hospital provided coverage for emergencies and certain medical procedures. The infrequent appearance of these medical neophytes sometimes caused problems. For example, one evening about eight o'clock, Dr. Long started an abdominal paracentesis (a tap of the peritoneal cavity to withdraw ascitic fluid) on Mrs. MacTeague. She had had this procedure regularly and tolerated it well. Dr. Long left the tubing draining into a basin under the bed. When the drainage stopped, the evening nurse called the intern to remove the neddle. The intern sauntered by the desk, asking, "What room?" He went into the room, withdrew the needle, left it and the tubing in the basin, and left the unit. He did not ask the patient's name, nor did he look at or write on the chart. A staff nurse did not accompany him. Later, Mrs. MacTeague complained of an unusual degree of abdominal pain, which required a call to her physician for a pain medication order.

Mrs. Kushner did not have cancer, but she was admitted to the Oncology Unit in an emergency. She had a history of congestive heart failure. As the researcher came into the unit one day, she heard a wail from the room, so she went in and saw that the patient was restrained, receiving oxygen, and restless. Mrs. Kushner asked the researcher to remove the restraints, but the researcher explained that she had just arrived on the unit and couldn't do that but would stay with her until one of the nurses could come in. When Vicki, a RN, came into the room, the patient became belligerent. Vicki was obviously annoyed at the patient and voiced relief that she was to be transferred to a medical unit. Vicki started to get the patient's belongings together, and the researcher went to the nurses' station.

A resident came by and told the head nurse that he wanted to examine Mrs. Kushner's chest but needed a nurse to hold her still, so Vicki went back into the room with him. When the resident came out to write on the chart, the head nurse told him that Mrs. Kushner had refused to have the brain scan he had ordered.

Upset, the resident asked, "How does a person with no medical background know what's good for her?"

Karen said, "You can't force her; she has a right to refuse."

The resident said, "In a courtroom they would say she's incompetent."

Karen responded, "There's the matter of injecting her with a radioisotope before the scan. Without her consent, in a courtroom they could cry assault and battery!" The resident did not seem satisfied. Karen turned and asked the listening researcher's opinion.

Her response was, "How could she even cooperate with a brain scan when she's in restraints and has to be held just to have her chest examined?" There was no further discussion, and Mrs. Kushner was soon transferred to a medical unit.

Mr. Horowitz, who had a colostomy and metastasis to the kidney and other sites, was known to the staff from previous admissions. This hospitalization was lengthy, and he was getting progressively worse. He was a popular patient, having been president of the region's Ostomy Club. One day Mr. Horowitz fell in his room and sustained abrasions on his neck. An incident report was filled out, and the resident, who did not know the patient or the attending physicians, was called to check him for injury and sign the report. A nurse said that the resident leafed through the *Physician's Desk Reference* and decided upon an antiseptic solution to be applied to the abrasions. The hospital pharmacy had to special-order the antiseptic, and by the time it arrived, two days later, the abrasions had almost healed. The nurse asked Dr. Thomas if the patient still needed it, and he said no, but the patient had incurred a totally unnecessary cost.

Medical students from a school in a nearby state had for some time received part of their clinical training on the general medical or surgical wards at Charles Hospital. Because of Charles' new affiliation with the state medical school, the nurses asked Dr. Fisher if medical students would be assigned to EH II when they started their clinical training the following year. Speaking to the supervisor, head nurse, and Annette, now an inservice education instructor, Dr. Fisher said, "Write or call State Medical Center and National Cancer Hospital and ask them how they deal with medical students on the ward." Then he moved on to some other business.

A few days later the situation was being discussed by the nurses. "It's not our responsibility to find out about medical students. Dr. Fisher should go to see Dr. Cassavetes, the director of medical education." The supervisor said she had sat on the issue, since she felt it was a matter to which Dr. Fisher, as medical director of the unit, should address himself, rather than delegate it to the nurses. Yet no one expressed this view to Dr. Fisher.

One day the supervisor and head nurse were discussing this issue with Dr. Thomas, who commented, "They ought to throw the g. d. medical students out of this hospital or redo the teaching program. It's terrible."

DOCTOR-DOCTOR CONFLICT

During the early months of the study, the researcher observed evidence of a problem between Dr. Long and Dr. Thomas, such as sarcastic remarks and disagreements about treatment, which they verbalized through the nurses. None of the nurses volunteered information about this, though they were heard commenting, usually sarcastically, about the relationship. Nurses as well as patients became involved in the problem between the two associates. For example, on rounds, a group went in to see Mr. Harrison, who had lung cancer with brain metastasis and was receiving radiation therapy. Dr. Long looked at the patient and the chart and asked Annette, the charge nurse that day, why the steroid was not being given. Annette looked at the chart and said, "There's no order for it."

Dr. Long said, "I gave a telephone order yesterday afternoon." Since Annette had been off at the time, she sent for Lisa, who came in looking a little flustered and explained the situation.

The afternoon before, Mr. Harrison had developed symptoms of a stroke (cerebrovascular accident). Lisa called Dr. Long, and when she described the patient's condition, he ordered a steroid to be given intravenously by slow drip. However, after the call Lisa realized that the patient didn't have an IV running, so she called the office back but got Dr. Thomas instead. She explained Mr. Harrison's situation to him. Dr. Thomas told her not to give the steroid or start the IV, and she followed Dr. Thomas' orders. However, since Lisa had not written Dr. Long's first order on the chart as a verbal order, she didn't write Dr. Thomas' counter-order, either. Therefore none of the events that had transpired became part of the patient's record.

Dr. Long was sitting at Mr. Harrison's bedside as he listened to this explanation and said, "Well, that's a difference of opinion about philosophy of treatment." He didn't say anything more and didn't order the steroid at that point.

The patient lived only a few more days. It was a complicated situation for the nurses because Mr. Harrison was estranged from his wife, and a girlfriend had been visiting him. But when his condition worsened, the wife and family started coming more frequently, so the girlfriend had to call before she came and ask the staff if other visitors were present.

There were many other examples of the two associates' philosophic differences about treatment, and Dr. Thomas had no qualms about mentioning his disagreement with Dr. Long to the nurses. One day on rounds he told them to read a medical journal article, indicating that he agreed with the philosophy and concepts put forth by the author. During the course of the research, members of the nursing staff made numerous unsolicited comments regarding their perception that Dr. Long treated patients too aggressively and too long. Though Dr. Thomas did not specify a passage from the article, one significant section stated:

> there is no need to prolong a useless and tragic life by forced feeding or giving antibiotics to frustrate bronchial pneumonia, the traditional friend of the hopelessly ill or the aged. It is inhuman to drag the dying patient to radiation therapy, to transfuse him repeatedly or to give massive doses of toxic chemotherapy to relieve one tiny facet of an intolerable existence, thereby dragging it out for a few more agonizing days or weeks. That is the science without the humanity of medicine [1].

Finally, the researcher asked several of the nurses about the situation. Lisa indicated that nurses and patients were very much caught up in it:

> The two partners don't agree on many things. One starts an IV and heavy medications, and the next day the other one stops the order. Do they want me to say to the patient, "Push, Push," or "I know how you feel if you don't want to get up"? Patients are often passive and don't realize this is happening. This floor basically avoids how we're going to deal with the patient.

But Libby, another RN, said, "They're so sick [the patients], they don't know what's going on." The supervisor cited an example of overt hostility between the doctors in the presence of patients, when Dr. Long had commented to the nurses that Dr. Thomas had no compassion for these patients. Mildred, who liked Dr. Thomas, had felt compelled to leave the room.

The nurses explained that patients tended to prefer one doctor or the other. "If they like Long, they don't like Thomas, and vice versa." Some of Dr. Long's patients had very positive things to say about him, such as, "He's a doll"; "I wish you were my doctor all the time"; or "I've been under this good doctors care for a year."

The Divorce

The strained relationship between Drs. Thomas and Long culminated in severance of the "partnership." In October, during a nursing staff meeting, Dr. Long stuck his head in the door of the conference room, and looking at the head nurse, said nonchalantly, "I want you to know that Dr. Thomas is no longer with the practice. Since I'll be working alone, you'll be seeing me at odd hours." He explained that Dr. Thomas might go into private practice but that he would have to apply for staff privileges as an independent practitioner.

Later, the researcher asked the head nurse, "Wasn't that announcement a surprise to the nurses? No one seemed to react."

Karen replied, "It was like he dropped a bomb." The head nurse and supervisor had thought the doctors were partners, but now they said Dr. Thomas wanted everyone in the hospital to know that he had been fired; Dr. Long had come to his house on a Sunday and hand-delivered a letter severing his contract. Dr. Thomas told the nurses that Dr. Long had had the locks changed in the office so that his former associate couldn't get in. None of the patients were given the choice of going with Dr. Thomas, they were simply told that he was no longer with the practice.

A great deal of moral support went to Dr. Thomas, who stayed in touch with three of the registered nurses while he set up his practice and waited to be given medical staff privileges. One nurse explained:

> He's starting from scratch. He's about thirty-five, and that's late to be starting out. He has nothing. He went directly from military service to work for Dr. Long. He'll need referrals and consultations from other physicians, but it will be hard because Dr. Fisher, as chief, gets all the oncology consultations, and Dr. Green is chief of hematology and gets all those consultations.

Dr. Green offered to give Dr. Thomas some duplicate equipment from his office laboratory. He made the offer through Karen, who told Dr. Thomas. Dr. Green asked Karen what kind of a person Dr. Thomas was, and Karen's response was, "He's bright, level, direct, and hurt over the way the association with Dr. Long was broken off."

The researcher had lunch one day in the cafeteria with Karen and Dr.

Thomas, who spoke about the legal severance of his contract. "I let my mouthpiece [lawyer] do the talking. I also put my office announcement card right down on J. C.'s [Jesus Christ] desk." He explained that Dr. Long had been getting a chemotherapeutic drug free from the manufacturer "by the load," supposedly for indigent patients. Dr. Thomas told the company representative that he too should get a supply of the drug for the indigent patients in his new practice. As a result, neither doctor was to get any.

Later, the researcher asked the head nurse how the rest of the nursing staff had reacted to the situation and was told that at first, nobody could believe that Dr. Long would fire Dr. Thomas. The general consensus was that it was unfair, but they knew Dr. Thomas had been unhappy working with Dr. Long. "And you could see it—contradictory orders day after day," the head nurse commented. She added that most of the people on the unit felt a loss when Dr. Thomas wasn't there for a month.

While the severance of the doctors' relationship lessened one source of the nurses' role strain, it added another. The head nurse commented:

> Now with Dr. Long—I wouldn't call it a neglect of patients, but one man taking care of this many patients is too much of a load. I have to call the office during the day about orders he probably would have written correctly if he had been less tired. His follow-up on IVs and electrolytes and things like that, which he used to keep up with, creates a monitoring problem for the nurses. You're really like babysitting. You have to watch the lab slips when they come in. I feel it's an imposition on my time because I should be doing nursing things.

The researcher asked if Karen thought she was doing a lot of physician-assisting tasks. "Oh yes. That's what he wants. He's asked me many times to work for him." Karen added that she told him she liked the hospital atmosphere and "I don't like his philosophy of treating patients."

The evening-shift nurses were also under more strain because Dr. Long sometimes made rounds in the evening. When one nurse called him regarding an incorrect suppository order, he laughed and said, "Did I write that?"

Nurses covered for Dr. Long as they did for the others, so that no harm from incorrect orders would come to a patient, but they also said that Long would be the first to call the nursing office with a complaint about something they had done or omitted to do. They resented this but didn't confront him about it.

As Dr. Thomas began admitting patients and building up a practice, several of the nurses let the researcher know. As his practice built up, they cheered for him. A government installation in a nearby city was discontinuing its outpatient cancer treatment program and since Dr. Thomas was known there, a large number of the patients were referred to him. "Wait until Dr. Long hears about that!" said the head nurse.

When the researcher got the opportunity, she asked the two physicians about the situation. Dr. Thomas said:

> There was a fundamental philosophic difference between me and my former associate. We had entirely different approaches to the care of patients with malignant disease and how an office should be run and how employees should be treated. Enough said.

The researcher continued, "Did it bother you that you were board-certified and your employer was not?"

Dr. Thomas replied, "It didn't bother me, but it bothered my former employer tremendously."

The researcher asked, "Isn't there a dilemma between expanding new treatment horizons through research and allowing death with dignity?"

"Yes, there is," replied Dr. Thomas. "But there are guidelines of study groups to follow, such as the regional Cooperative Oncology Group."

The researcher suggested to Dr. Thomas that perhaps the termination of the relationship was for the better. He replied: "I'm sure it was. I'm weary running all over the place, but at least I don't have to face having my work undone or having the patient caught in the middle."

"What about your present relationship with Dr. Long?" the researcher asked.

"He doesn't even exist," replied Dr. Thomas.

After the "divorce," the researcher rarely saw Dr. Thomas on rounds because he was admitting few patients. When she did see him, his manner with his own patients was attentive and nonabrasive, but he continued to make sarcastic comments about his former employer. One day in the nurses' station he heard that Dr. Long had admitted Mrs. Georgetti for further radiation therapy. Mrs. Georgetti, whom Dr. Thomas knew from his former practice, had had brain metastasis. "Full speed ahead. She needs a feeding tube and a tracheostomy," commented Dr. Thomas sarcastically to the nurses, indicating again his dissension with Dr. Long's philosophy of treatment.

When the researcher asked Dr. Long about the severance of the partnership, he replied:

> I was in oncology practice for five years before I hired Dr. Thomas three years ago, first part-time, then full-time. I was warned about him before I hired him. People trained in hematology don't know anything about oncology. They just get into it. He was too sarcastic.

The researcher asked if he was going to get another associate. "Perhaps in time, when I get over my divorce," said Dr. Long.

Timing of Rounds

In the beginning of the research year, Drs. Long and Thomas alternated daily rounds to the same group of patients. Dr. Thomas was very predictable, arriving about eight in the morning, moving through rounds, charting at a regular pace, and leaving the unit promptly. Dr. Long, as one of the nurses said, might arrive at any time, see some of the patients, leave the unit, come back, then leave again, so that rounds stretched out over a considerable period of time. Generally, Drs. Thomas and Long wrote orders and progress notes on the patients' charts at the bedside, sitting on the bed or in a chair. Narcotic orders had to be rewritten every forty-eight hours, whereas there was a seven-day renewal policy for other drugs.

Dr. Fisher was predictable in that the staff knew what hour he would come in, but his hours varied on different days of the week to fit his office hours. For example, on Tuesdays, for a good part of the year, he arrived for rounds about five in the morning, because his office hours started at seven o'clock. He would caution the patients the day before, "I'll be coming in tomorrow with a flashlight." The hospital would be dark when he arrived, and most patients were sleeping. He would use a flashlight to check the patients, or, if all the occupants of a room were his patients, he would turn on the overhead light behind the patient's bed.

Dr. Fisher's early rounds didn't seem to bother his patients', nor did they seem to resent being awakened. Catherine, one of the night RNs, liked making rounds during the night. She said it gave her a chance to learn, to get to know the patients better, and to see the manner in which Dr. Fisher related to the patients, which she described as "terrific." Catherine added, "I don't care how the doctors treat me as long as they're good to their patients." She regretted that she couldn't go on rounds with Dr. Fisher every night he came in, "but so many of the patients start waking up and are uncomfortable at that time."

On one occasion, Catherine left the unit to get some medication for Dr. Fisher to give a patient intravenously. He came to the desk and said to the researcher, "What are you doing here at this ungodly hour? Where's Catherine?" The researcher told him that Catherine had gone downstairs to get a drug for him. He remarked, "Catherine's a good girl. I wish she were on this unit all the time." Nurses had no control over the timing of rounds, although their occurrence, along with the subsequent changes in medical orders for patients, was an important consideration in the organization of work on the unit. Moreover, staff sometimes experienced greater time pressure than usual. For example, one day Dr. Long unexpectedly came to make rounds in midafternoon. A surgeon who happened to be on the unit commented that it was an unusual time for him. "Routine is dull," Dr. Long replied. The nurses grimaced because it was close to the three o'clock change-of-shift report, and they knew that all the new orders would have to be taken care of before they left.

A marked change in the timing of rounds occurred after the split between Drs. Long and Thomas. On certain days of the week, Dr. Long made rounds late in the evening. He explained that he had leased his office space for certain hours and couldn't change them. However, since he didn't have an associate, he had to manage office hours at two locations and visits to two hospitals, as well as his other professional activities. He rarely took a day off, but when he did, an internist covered for him, usually unannounced. Once he stated, "Every once in awhile I feel like a vacation, but then I wake up in the morning and realize it's impossible."

Dr. Long arrived as late as ten o'clock on some nights. The head nurse commented:

> He expects the three-to-eleven nurses to make rounds with him and assist him with certain procedures, but they don't have any extra help on three-to-eleven because his hours have changed. They don't have a ward clerk either for taking all the orders off the charts. One night he wrote orders on fourteen charts.

It was the researcher's observation that the evening staff paid little attention to Dr. Long when he arrived late unless they had a specific request or problem about a patient. The staff continued their usual work, while he made rounds by himself and asked for help if he needed it.

In general, patients did not overtly object to the late rounds. However, some of the patients did not see him, since they had been medicated and were asleep, hopefully, for the night. Though he didn't always wake sleeping patients, he did write progress notes on their charts, and as the staff reminded the researcher, that proved, for billing purposes, that the doctor had been there.

Some patients did object to the late night rounds. One day, when the researcher went into Mr. Donahoo's room, his wife and daughter were there. They had brought his clothes to the hospital because they understood that he was to be discharged that day. However, there was no discharge order on the chart, and the head nurse's attempts to reach Dr. Long had been unsuccessful for two hours.

Mr. Donahoo was angry. He said of Dr. Long: "He was in here last night at eleven o'clock, and the night before at ten-thirty. Now he can't be reached. What kind of a way is that to operate?" When the head nurse finally contacted Dr. Long, he told her that Mr. Donahoo had to stay until he came in to check him. Mr. Donahoo was not discharged for several more days.

Some of the nursing staff were sympathetic to Dr. Long when he made late rounds and was obviously fatigued. One Friday night he left the unit at nine o'clock, saying he hadn't had lunch or dinner and still had rounds to make at Overhill Hospital, which was about one-half hour away. He giddily grabbed an apple off the desk on his way out.

One night, Dr. Long arrived for rounds at quarter to nine. He picked out the charts of his fourteen patients and started making rounds by himself. About nine, he went into Mrs. MacTeague's room and told the seventy-four-year-old that he wanted to do a paracentesis. Mrs. MacTeague had been having this procedure done regularly for about three years. That night she told Dr. Long she didn't want it done; she was tired enough from getting a blood transfusion. He said OK. Mrs. MacTeague said to the researcher, "He's my sweetie." She motioned to Dr. Long and whispered that the newly admitted patient in the opposite bed was Dr. Thomas' patient.

Loudly, Dr. Long replied, "Well, we won't hold that against her."

Mrs. MacTeague was a lonely woman who welcomed a greeting or a chat. She said, "Dr. Thomas came in to see my roommate and didn't even say hello to me. I never did anything to him."

Three nights earlier, Mrs. MacTeague had wept as she told the researcher that her only child, a daughter, "took her own life at the age of fifty-two," a few years previously. A long history of marital dischord and a recent diagnosis of Parkinsonism had been contributing factors. Mrs. MacTeague's husband had died six months before the daughter, while Mrs. MacTeague was hospitalized for cancer of the ovary. After her husband's death she had sold her home and given her daughter a large portion of the sale price. "My son-in-law took me in," she said, indicating that the situation was less than ideal because of the memory of her daughter's problems, but "at least I have a home." The son-in-law and his girlfriend, both in their sixties, were her only visitors. She sobbed as she said how he missed her daughter. A few nights later, after Dr. Long finished writing on Mrs. MacTeague's chart, he looked up from the bedside and loudly said to the researcher, "Her daughter commited suicide, you know." The researcher merely nodded. "Oh, she told you," added Dr. Long.

Mrs. MacTeague had been admitted with a disturbance in equilibrium, which was attributed to brain metastasis. Her symptoms cleared with radiation therapy and a different course of chemotherapy. She noted that her hair was falling out; "this will be the third time," she said. A few months later, she was admitted again, totally disoriented with organic brain syndrome. Her son-in-law was unable to care for her any longer, and she was awaiting nursing home placement as the researcher was concluding data collection.

Nurses' Attitudes About Medical Treatment

There was a consensus among the registered nurses that Dr. Long treated patients too aggressively, too long, although the researcher did observe exceptions. The head nurse said that when she spoke to Dr. Long about this, his response was that the nurses didn't see how his office patients responded to treatment. Annette's view changed over the course of time. Initially, she told the researcher:

> There's a lot of frustration on this floor. Sometimes you think you're in the middle as the nurse between the doctor and the patient. From working here you get an instinct that a patient's life is coming to an end. . . . there's an instinct . . . and from working with the patients you know that if everything was stopped, tests and all that, they would be satisfied. You see them being trucked down to X-Ray and over to the next state for EMIs and all unnecessary things and nine times out of ten you're right.

The researcher asked Annette how she knew she was right. "Because they die in a short time," she replied.

"What about the one out of ten?" asked the researcher. "Some do bounce back; some do surprise you," she said; "but there's a lack of openness with the patient about the patient's present state."

After Annette was transferred to the Inservice Education Department and had been off the unit for a few months, she made this contribution at a staff conference:

> You change your ideas when you leave the floor. I'm more aware of the will to survive since we've had the experience of a close family friend with a brain tumor. She's down on EH I. Your attitude becomes, "Give me what there is. There's nothing else."

The first time Mildred Hayes ever heard Dr. Long give a prognosis since the opening of the unit was when he told Marge Holland's family in February that she had a one- to two-month prognosis. Marge, a forty-seven-year-old legal secretary, had liver metastasis subsequent to malignant melanoma. During this five-week hospitalization, Marge failed to respond to hepatic artery chemotherapy and grew progressively weaker, with jaundice, bleeding tendencies, and other signs of liver failure. Her abdomen was markedly enlarged with ascites, and her legs and ankles were edematous. Marge had continually voiced her desire to go home after the unsuccessful chemotherapy. However, she developed septicemia, and Dr. Long started her on an antibiotic research protocol. Finally, on a Sunday, Dr. Long told Marge and her family that she could go home the following Wednesday, and he wrote on the chart, "for terminal care." Her sisters were going to care for her. On Monday and Tuesday Dr. Long ordered more lab tests and platelet transfusions for Marge, who was becoming increasingly confused and afraid that she had been incontinent of urine and feces. On Wednesday, her mother and brother came to take her home. Her lips and mouth were bloody when she left, but she knew she was going home, and she knew that she had arrived. She died in her bed six hours after discharge from the hospital.

The nurses wondered what difference the platelet transfusions could make, when what Marge wanted was a few more days at home. The researcher asked the group why they thought Marge, or her family, had consented to an antibiotic research protocol that took twelve days. "Wouldn't another drug have done the job and gotten her home sooner?" The consensus was yes, but one nurse said, "Instead of telling patients the study takes ten to twelve days, Long probably says a few days or some other vague term."

Nurses explained that patients often consented to treatment they didn't really want because of their faith in the doctor. One nurse added: "If Long gets one patient to respond to a research protocol, it gets his hopes up, and he tries the same thing on everybody with a similar condition."

After the "divorce," Dr. Long continued to treat patients in what nurses thought was an overaggressive manner. They were intimately caught up in this conflict because they were obliged to carry out the doctor's orders for treatment. A night nurse, after getting a report that Mrs. Edwards, who was semicomatose and diaphoretic, was on tube feedings and IVs, said, "Doesn't look like she'll last the night. But to the end, he'll pump stuff in. Why does he do that?" The patient died eleven days later.

Ted, the nurse who conducted the rap sessions for the nursing staff, listened to staff verbalize this conflict on many occasions. His conclusion was that "Dr. Long seems to be a major denier."

Occasionally, a nurse would make a comment to Dr. Long about his mode of treatment. Mr. Leonard, an eighty-year-old man, who was hospitalized for about two months, was a favorite of the nurses; his patience and charm had captivated them. When he was thought to be ready for discharge, Dr. Long decided that Mr. Leonard needed another course of radiation therapy. He already had a contracted bladder and many urinary problems from bladder involvement with the previous radiation treatment, and there was much consternation among the nurses that at his age, he should receive another course of treatment. "He should refuse," said Ellen, a graduate nurse on the evening shift. "Tell his daughter she should refuse," she pleaded.

Mr. Leonard did complete the second course of radiation therapy and improved sufficiently to be discharged to his daughter's care with some homemaker assistance. Before a week was up, however, he was readmitted, severely deteriorated, dehydrated, and disoriented. Mildred Hayes was in charge of the unit when Dr. Long came in. He asked Mildred what she thought he should do about Mr. Leonard. Mildred replied by asking him what difference it would make what she thought; he would go ahead and treat Mr. Leonard as he saw fit anyway. Contrary to Mildred's and the staff's expectations, Dr. Long did not order a urinary catheter, IV fluids, antibiotics, and other measures. Mr. Leonard was given only basic comfort measures and died the next night, with Ellen holding him and the aides giving him care.

Another time, Mr. Edwards came from Southside Hospital in the southern part of the state to be under Dr. Long's care. He had lung cancer but also had pulmonary emphysema. After an episode of chest pain during the night, his EKG showed evidence of a myocardial infarction. Dr. Long told the nurses to keep him on bed rest. Dr. Long called someone at Southside and stated that every time he attempted to treat Mr. Edwards (with radiation), he "fills up; he's so filled with emphysema that he doesn't have much tolerance." Dr. Long stated that he wanted to send Mr. Edwards back to Soutside to be nearer his family, but he wanted to be sure that Medicare permitted this type of transfer. On another occasion Medicare hadn't covered a patient's transfer back to Southside, and Charles had ended up paying the patient's bill as a service patient.

Although the nursing staff had much to say about what they regarded as Dr. Long's overaggressive medical treatment, the researcher heard only one such comment made within hearing of a patient who was receiving such treatment. Mrs. Austin was admitted for the fourth time during the research year with extensive metastasis from breast cancer. She was markedly "Cushingoid" from steroid therapy and, despite the fact that she was in extreme back pain, requiring narcotics every two hours, she wanted to go home. However, she developed septicemia with high fever and periods of confusion. She was also depressed, covering herself entirely with a bed sheet and not bothering to wear her wig. She refused to be fitted for a spinal brace that Dr. Long had ordered, stating to the bracemaker that it was a waste of money. She was treated with intravenous antibiotics and steroids, received platelet transfusions, and had a nasogastric tube connected to suction. Failing to respond, Mrs. Austin became increasingly disoriented and required restraints to keep her from pulling out the IV tubing. The researcher walked into the room as Libby, the RN "grandmother" of the unit, was adding another IV antibiotic. "This is a sin; it's nothing but a waste of money," Libby said.

Mrs. Austin died the next day. The nurses said Dr. Long commented that she wouldn't have died if Charles Hospital stocked the kind of replacement thyroid hormone she required. Dr. Long had a reputation for denying that cancer was a cause of patients' deaths. One of the administrative staff at Charles commented to the researcher, "Oh, you're on the Oncology Unit. Dr. Long says nobody ever dies of cancer. I see him at Cancer Society meetings."

MEDICAL RESEARCH

When the researcher started data collection, Dr. Long was conducting a study on a pain medication for a pharmaceutical company. It was a double-blind study, managed from the pharmacy, in which patients received either 10 mg of morphine or an equivalent dose of a research drug. A small article from a national newspaper on the bulletin board described the new drug as "nonaddictive, relieves pain longer than morphine, there's no dizziness, nausea or hallucinatory effect."

Patients on the study were identified as being on pain "protocol." Dr. Long determined who should be on the protocol, and the patient or a family member had to give consent. If the patient did not get relief from the medication, the order was changed to a conventional pain relief medication. The researcher observed that there was no systematic assessment of patients' pain relief in the study, nor were any special nursing records or even regular records kept on the chart about the patient's pain or its relief. None of the unit's nurses had read the pain research proposal, though all the RNs and LPNs were involved in the study by virtue of the fact that they gave the drug, and in the usual course of nursing care were supposed to observe and record the effects and side effects of drugs.

Since Dr. Thomas was Dr. Long's associate at the time of the study, he naturally saw all the patients on protocol. One day the researcher heard a patient moaning. The group on rounds with Dr. Thomas went to Mrs. Kaiser's bed in the alcove of a three-bed room. Two days earlier the moaning patient had had a decompressive laminectomy for spinal metastasis with spinal chord compression and now she had "acute brain syndrome." Her eyes were open, but she did not have reflexes—when Dr. Thomas brought his hand down swiftly, stopping short just before Mrs. Kaiser's open eyes, she showed no response. She was restless and thrashing around, crying, "Buddy, I love you" and, "Mommy, Mommy, help me." The nurses said she had exhibited the same behavior on the evening and night shifts and that during visiting hours the evening before, she hadn't recognized her family.

Sitting by the bedside and leafing through the chart, Dr. Thomas noted that Mrs. Kaiser was on protocol for pain. Referring to Dr. Long he said to the nurses, "How can he put a patient who's irrational on a double-blind study? He must be desperate for patients at the end of the study."

One evening Dr. Long asked if the researcher was interested in working for him as a research assistant on a pain project. He asked what salary she was making in her part-time nursing employment. When she gave a rough estimate, Dr. Long said, "I can make it worthwhile for you." The researcher asked Dr. Long how he monitored the pain study that was being done since she didn't see any record of patient response on the charts. He said, "It's in the computer."

The researcher again sought clarification by asking, "But how did you decide if relief was obtained? From nurses' notes? From patients' statements?"

Dr. Long replied, "I asked patients and recorded it. But nobody was aware that I was doing it." The nursing staff had told the researcher that a staff person from Dr. Long's office had come to the hospital to Xerox the patients' medication Kardexes, which showed the dose and amount given.

Dr. Long went on to explain to the researcher that he had a research lab at a university medical center in a nearby state. "I had $300,000 in grants last year." That startled the researcher, and she laughingly asked how much he pocketed of that. "Not much," replied Dr. Long; "I put it into research. I have a full-time technician, but she can't do the full-time pain study because she can't give medications, though she is more competent than some who are giving them."

The researcher responded by saying that she was really interested in the hospice movement—one seemed so much needed in the area.

Dr. Long replied: "I've looked into that, including federal grants. It would take three years to get off the ground in this state. It wouldn't go over anyway. Doctors are too economic-minded to treat patients without third-party payment."

Dr. Long had asked many nurses to work for him on the new pain project. He asked a particular nurse several times, but this nurse told the researcher:

> I don't like his tactics. Why does he convince these patients so strongly? He says to some, "If all you would do is eat, you would go home." Sometimes I believe that some of the patients do believe him. Maybe they get back to the denial phase.
>
> I really don't think he's honest—I really don't. He's hard to confront—he can become nasty. He ends up making you feel like a fool. He's made people cry in their day. He has the power to save lives. He kids and jokes about being called "J. C." He's a hard-sell salesman. I told him, "I'm leery of you." But you can't insult the man. I told him I was a "career" nurse, and I wanted to get a master's degree. He said, "I'll pay for a master's degree in pharmacology." I said, "I want one in nursing."

In June Dr. Long finally succeeded in hiring a nurse who had been a head nurse on another Charles unit.

One afternoon in the late spring, Dr. Long came to the unit nattily dressed and carrying under his arm a bound volume, which he held up for the nurses to see. He had been to a seminar to present the results of the pain protocol study. The researcher happened to be at the desk and asked Dr. Long if she could borrow the volume. Dr. Long declined to lend it, explaining that it was still privileged information and belonged to the drug company. The researcher asked if there would be a copy in the medical library. He said, "You're kidding. They don't pay one bit of attention to my other publications."

The researcher was told by a key informant that it took the pharmacy staff twenty minutes to set up a patient for the pain study. The informant added:

> Long was supposedly the one to be following the patients from the progress notes. There was no specific tool to record the patients' response. It was what nurses told him about whether or not the drug helps the patient.
>
> It occurred to me that if this is the way drug companies get medications on the market, it's a very loose process, a very sad way. It's about as loose as anything could possibly be.

Patients with cancer have a high incidence of septicemia. In fact, infection, precipitated by the underlying tumor, is a major cause of death in cancer patients. A second drug company-sponsored research project conducted by Dr. Long involved an antibiotic given intravenously to patients with septicemia and other infections. Patients of Dr. Thomas and Dr. Fisher, on the other hand, were receiving investigational drugs as part of studies that were approved and sponsored by federal government research agencies. Information necessary for the observation of these patients was kept in a drawer at the nurses' station.

Dr. Long's antibiotic study required monitoring certain laboratory tests; wound, sputum, and urine cultures, as well as twenty-four-hour urinalyses, had to be repeated at regular intervals. Apparently, when Dr. Long initially explained the drug and obtained the patients' consent, he did not tell them that they would incur the extra costs of monitoring the drug's effects. Some of the tests, though not all, would probably have been ordered if the patients were treated with another antibiotic.

Frances, the supervisor, believed it was unfair that the patients should incur these extra charges without their consent. In this instance, she acted as the patients' advocate and pursued the issue until it was agreed that the drug company would bear the expense for the monitoring. After that, samples sent to the lab were marked "Infection Protocol," and charges were billed to the drug company. An informant said:

> The drug company research I have real questions about. Patients are told they will get the drug free but not that there's additional lab work and perhaps additional days in the hospital. So it's not just the effects they should be informed about, but the costs also. It could cause patients to run out of their insurance benefits earlier.

The informant explained that approval for research drugs was supposed to be granted by a Research Committee composed of six to eight physicians, one nurse (the Oncology Unit supervisor), one pharmacist, and one representative from hospital administration. But the informant added:

> Many of the doctors don't come to the meetings, and administration has been remiss in not having a representative present. They really should come

to learn what's going on in this hospital. The proposal goes to each committee member but a lot of them only initial it and return it. The grant money from the pharmaceutical companies goes to the physician personally, not to the pharmacy or lab. If third-party payers ever found out they're paying for certain pharmaceutical companies to investigate new drugs . . . .

Doctors avoided interaction with each other on investigational drug policies, but the nurses fostered this attitude by acting as intermediaries in doctors' disputes. For example, one day the head nurse was in the conference room explaining the use of an infusion pump to a new nurse. The pump (a metered drip device used to regulate the flow rate of potent solutions) was to be used in administering an investigational drug to one of Dr. Fisher's patients, a nineteen-year-old with embryonal-teratocarcinoma of the testicle with metastasis to retroperitoneal nodes and lungs. (During the year, three young men were admitted for such treatment.)

Dr. Long, overhearing a conversation about the drug at the nurses' station, looked into the conference room and said, "I hate to be paranoid but . . . ." Apparently, at one time he had been denied permission to give the drug in the way Dr. Fisher intended to give it, and also the policy was that nurses could not prepare or hang IVs of investigational drugs. The supervisor was consulted as well as Dr. Fisher, "who was really ticked off" at this interference with his plans. It was decided that the protocol for the investigational drug had to be cleared through the P&T Committee (Pharmacy and Therapeutics), as well as the Research Committee.

The task of expediting this fell to the supervisor, who with the head nurse, spent much of the day on this issue. Dr. Green, chairman of P&T, told the supervisor that Dr. Fisher should get together with Dr. Long and Dr. Thomas about investigational oncology drugs since the P&T Committee was not all that familiar with them. The committee wanted the Oncology Department, headed by Dr. Fisher, to submit unified requests for review, rather than receiving requests from the individual doctors on the oncology service.

Frances had to meet with Dr. Fisher to resolve the issue at six-thirty the next morning after he finished rounds. Afterward, Frances said:

It's clear that Dr. Fisher doesn't want a meeting with Dr. Long on this. He doesn't want a confrontation. Dr. Fisher says he's going to write a book on how non-problems become problems, and that the best thing to do with Dr. Long is to ignore him.

This was possible for Dr. Fisher, since he rarely made rounds at the same time as Dr. Long, but the nurses had to deal with Dr. Long every day and were unable to ignore him.

The P&T Committee turned down the request to permit nurses to mix and hang the drug; either Dr. Fisher had to prepare and hang it himself, or an intern or resident had to come to the unit to do it. Dr. Fisher told the nurses to write to other hospitals and find out their policies on nurses administering investigational drugs.

After the episode about the investigational drug, the head nurse commented, "Management is no easy job. There are so many kinds of interactions that you get involved in."

The supervisor commented:

You might find this difficult to believe, but sometimes I find Dr. Long easier to deal with than Dr. Fisher. His manner is different but just as difficult. Long rants and raves and spreads the situation all over the hospital, but Dr. Fisher won't deal with the problems that he's supposed to deal with as director of the unit; and that is just as bad, if not worse.

The researcher asked a group of staff nurses how they perceived Dr. Fisher's relationship to the other doctors. One responded:

There's no communication flow. The doctors go their independent ways. Dr. Terwilliger from the Radiation Therapy Department suggested that they all meet to review interesting cases, but that went over like a lead balloon. The doctors don't communicate with each other.

When the opportunity arose, the researcher asked Dr. Fisher if he, as director of the unit, exerted any control over the admitting physicians. He replied, "I'm director of the unit because when it was founded I was the only one board-certified. I don't exert control over other doctors. If there's a general floor problem, I grab all the doctors to discuss it."

The researcher asked, "What about the problem of informed consent and research?"

"You can play around with him as long as you like," was Dr. Fisher's reply. (He was referring to Dr. Long but was not open to further discussion.)

The nurses volunteered the information that when Dr. Fisher and Dr. Green were partners, Dr. Green had to force himself to start on rounds, when it was his turn. Since Dr. Green was basically a hematologist, his specialty was with diseases such as leukemia (liquid cancers rather than solid tumors). The nurses observed that Dr. Green found it increasingly difficult to deal with fistulas, gaping wounds, ostomies, infections, and the other complications seen in patients with solid cancers. Nurses explained to the researcher that after the Fisher-Green partnership broke up, Dr. Green admitted very few patients to the Oncology Unit. Nurses said that the two physicians were not on speaking terms.

The researcher asked Dr. Fisher, "Was the breakup of the professional association with your former partner an amicable one?" She sensed some resistance.

"Is that relevant?" asked Dr. Fisher.

The researcher said, "From what I've seen here it could lead to another question for exploration."

"What's that?"

"Whether the stresses of oncology practice make it difficult for a partnership to exist. Is oncology an essentially lonely field?"

Dr. Fisher replied, "Dr. Green was not a trained oncologist. There was a different philosophy about workload; I was just overworked, that's all."

When the researcher asked Dr. Long about his view of the stresses of an oncology practice on physician relationships, he replied:

> It is lonely by the nature of the disease, and they get at each other. I'm not on the Tumor Board yet because Dr. Fisher's tried to keep me out. This is a business. Doctors get paid for each research protocol they send in—each report.

Dr. Long went on to explain that lack of cooperation among physicians was to be expected since doctors in relatively new practices are in competition with each other for patients. He thought that only time would resolve the problems. On another occasion, Dr. Long revealed to the researcher, "Physicians are prima donnas. There are lots of jealousies among doctors in this field. It's very competitive. Even at University Medical Center oncologists don't like each other and don't cover for each other."

TREATMENT PHILOSOPHIES

Since involvement with bioethical issues, such as prolongation of life, the use of investigational drugs, and informed consent, is an intimate facet of an oncology practice, the researcher queried each physician on his philosophy of treatment.

Dr. Fisher stated his belief that cancer should be treated like any other disease and that the degree of aggression should be the same as for any other disease. "My goal is to build up self-esteem in patients so they can be their own decision maker. Cancer destroys their sense of independence. It also destroys their thought processes." Noting that there are emotional differences between patients, Dr. Fisher said he believed the doctor must give every bit of emotional support needed. "If patients want another doctor's opinion, I am glad to make an appointment. I have contacts at major university treatment centers in two different cities," he added.

Dr. Thomas said he believed that the doctor should:

> help patients as much as he can, but let them die with dignity. Patients should die without being uncomfortable, and families should be protected from unnecessary strain. If death is the inevitable outcome in three to four weeks, why go for broke and saddle the patient and family with extra grief?

The researcher asked, "What if the family wants everything done?"

He replied, "Respect the family's wishes in everything reasonable except heroic measures such as ventilators and resuscitation." With regard to specific forms of treatment, such as intravenous antibiotics or home care, he responded, "It depends; each patient is considered individually. Home care is better than nursing home care, but this must be weighed for the individual."

Dr. Long said that cancer should be treated the same as any other disease. He added:

> The end point is palliation. You must establish rapport with the patient so that patients feel you're on their side. They feel that you're doing something. If left alone, a patient could linger for three to four months. The family feels better if you're trying to help them. You can tell if you have that rapport because patients trust you. If you don't have rapport, you see them going here and there for treatment.

Because many of the nurses seemed to be in conflict with the degree of aggressiveness of Dr. Long's treatment, the researcher attempted on several occasions to set up an appointment with him to further discuss his philosophy of treatment. One day, she jokingly blocked his exit from the nurses' station and asked him to leave fifteen to twenty minutes for her at the end of rounds. He said, "I have to be in the office by eleven o'clock."

The researcher said she could go to his office. "I want to give you the opportunity to respond to some issues that have been raised," she explained.

"I'll dictate a letter," he volunteered.

"They are philosophic questions," the researcher said.

"How can I discuss philosophic questions in twenty minutes? If Carter's proposal to put a cap on income goes through, I'll go into research." The researcher stated that she didn't understand the comment. "It takes away individual incentive and motivation of physicians. To put a ceiling on income, patients will be treated like herds of cattle. It would take away the art of medicine. I don't have time to see you."

Again the researcher said, "I can go to your office," but Dr. Long didn't respond. He was writing a history and physical on a patient, who, a nurse pointed out, hadn't arrived on the unit yet. Another nurse was at the desk preparing a medication for him to give.

When Dr. Long saw that the researcher was still there, he said, "I believe in prayer. Prayer and laetrile." Laughing, he continued, "If the FDA approves it, I'm going to do a controlled study on it." The researcher had difficulty getting Dr. Long to be serious, as did the staff nurses.

Resuscitation

During the year, a few patients died suddenly and unpredictably. In the absence of autopsy data, the doctors attributed these deaths to cardiac arrhythmias or massive embolic phenomena. There were no resuscitation attempts (code nine's) during the year. The researcher was told by the nursing staff that there was no specific policy about resuscitation. Apparently, not much thought had been given to this issue. Calling a code seemed to be a matter of individual nursing judgment. Mildred recalled four codes in three and a half years. The one she called involved a man who had been dressed to go home and had collapsed while walking from his bed to a wheelchair. "He was coded, but he died," said Mildred, adding that when she called Dr. Thomas to notify him that the resuscitation attempt was in progress, he asked her why she called it. He directed her to have the team stop its efforts if they were unsuccessful after seven minutes. Mildred said, "At that time Dr. Thomas said he wouldn't code anybody on EH II."

As the discussion continued, Mildred said, "I know where I'm at with Dr. Fisher—he'd never want a code." But the others disagreed pointing out that Mike Raup, a nineteen-year-old patient of Dr. Fisher's, was responding to treatment for cancer of the testicle. Mildred agreed she would call a code on him. A nurse pointed out that when Mrs. Brown was readmitted to another unit with liver metastasis, Dr. Fisher wrote on her chart, "Patient is a code candidate." He wrote this on the chart again when Mrs. Brown was transferred to the Intensive Care Unit with uncontrolled gastrointestinal bleeding. The head nurse told the group that Dr. Fisher felt it necessary to have a conference with the ICU nurses to explain his rationale and stressed that cancer is a chronic disease. The ICU nurses couldn't understand why anyone with cancer should be in the Intensive Care Unit, let alone be coded.

A staff nurse cited another example. Dr. Fisher had given a three-month prognosis for Flo Hamill when she was first admitted. After a course of radiation therapy, she showed slight improvement but had multiple metastatic sites and a great deal of pain. Dr. Fisher commented to the head nurse that he hoped no one would call a code on Flo. The head nurse said she didn't think anybody would, but no medical or nursing order was written on the chart or Kardex to this effect.

Mildred said, "I'm sure every one of Long's would get coded."

The head nurse replied, "I'm not so sure." She had just recently asked him if Mr. Kravitz should be coded if he arrested, and Dr. Long "shook his head emphatically no." Mr. Kravitz was forty-seven and had multiple myeloma and extensive metastasis.

Though nurses had the responsibility for deciding whether to initiate resuscitation attempts, they were not concerned about the lack of clarity in this policy, nor did any further clarification of policies with the physicians result from this discussion.

Dying Trajectories

It was the researcher's impression that it was difficult to predict an illness course for many of the patients. Some who were moribund on admission recovered sufficiently to be discharged; others showed improvement for brief periods, and some deteriorated rapidly after initially responding to treatment. The researcher asked the doctors if they could accurately predict a patient's death. Dr. Fisher replied, "Only within one week or a few days."

Dr. Thomas said, "Unpredictability is the nature of the disease; some will die on course, some won't."

Dr. Long had a more expansive response:

> That's the disease, and that's what third-party payers are so stupid about. They give a certain amount of days and then you're supposed to discharge a patient. You know when a patient has lung cancer and is expectorating blood that he can exsanguinate at any time. Yet I have had to discharge patients and that's happened to a few shortly after they went home.

> That's the disease, and when you see a lot of patients, you know what to expect.

PHYSICIAN-NURSE RELATIONSHIPS

Doctors' views of nurses and nursing were obtained from their statements and inferred from their actions. Clearly, doctors had the positions of power on the unit, but Dr. Fisher told the researcher that "nurses are professionals with a different expertise." When asked if he thought nurses had reservations about being more assertive in their relationships with doctors, he replied, "I like to feel that my ability to tolerate advice from people is a measure of my maturity."

Dr. Thomas stated: "I have a somewhat less traditional view of doctor-nurse relationships, especially with hospital nurses. You can't get along without the nurses."

When data collection started, a copy of a letter from Dr. Long to the director of nursing was posted on the bulletin board of the nurses' station, citing the improvement in nursing care since Karen Foster became the head nurse. The staff joked about it, saying they planned to tack it up each time he had a complaint. The supervisor thought Dr. Long's attitude change, which prompted the letter, came about because the nursing service was more willing to get involved with his drug research. An LPN told the researcher, "Dr. Long does compliment us; he tells patients the reason they're doing good is because they're getting good nursing care.''

Leaving a patient's bedside one day, the nurses told Dr. Long they couldn't carry out his verbal order since it was clearly in the medical purview and contrary to hospital policy. He commented loudly, ''I could never be a nurse. You can't do anything!''

While there were several indications that the traditional doctor-nurse game was not being played on this unit, in that doctors were more open to nurses' suggestions, the nurses' behavior pattern was largely that of deferring to doctors rather than of being the patient's advocate. For example, Mrs. Varney had had a hip pinning for a pathologic fracture. One day, when Dr. Thomas told Mrs. Varney that she would have to get out of bed for her own good, she started to cry, a reaction that was not surprising because Mrs. Varney did not want to move. After pulling back the covers to check her legs, Dr. Thomas wrote an order for physical therapy and reminded the nurses to use sandbags to keep Mrs. Varney's feet from rotating outward. Three RNs and one LPN were on rounds with him. The group stepped outside Mrs. Varney's closed curtain and Dr. Thomas said, ''Well, should we or should we not heparinize her? Let's take a straw vote. What do you think, Annette?''

As Annette began to give her opinion, with the others listening attentively, the researcher went behind the curtain to Mrs. Varney, who was still crying. The patient, who was large and heavy, asked some questions about how much weight-bearing and walking she would have to do. Clearly, she was afraid of another fracture and wanted to be lifted to a chair without making any effort herself. On her previous admission, the nurses had complained that Mrs. Varney didn't want to help herself and leaned so heavily on them that they were afraid they would be injured by her weight.

The group had moved to Mrs. Luckman's bed. Dr. Thomas asked her how many radiation treatments she had left. She said, ''None, and never again. I would never advise anybody to have them.'' Mrs. Luckman's daughter was sitting at her bedside. The doctor ordered Mrs. Luckman's morphine increased to every two hours, if necessary, for her rib and chest pain.

Next the group went to Loretta Walters, a very large, pretty, fifty-year-old woman who looked pale and weak. She told Dr. Thomas that her legs had felt extremely weak when she got up to sit in a chair. ''It's as if I have no control over them,'' Loretta said. Dr. Thomas pulled back the covers from the top to examine her legs. Because she was so large (280 pounds), the hospital gown came only to her hips. One of the nurses did attempt to pull the gown down, but the patient was exposed below the hips, and no one suggested to the doctor that he wait until they obtained a drape sheet for the patient. He asked her to do straight leg raising. When Loretta put her left foot down, it went into an involuntary tremor.

Dr. Thomas said, "Well, we might as well let the neurosurgeons have a look at you. Everyone else has." To the nurses he remarked, "She must have the record for the most consultations of anyone on the ward."

Another day, after the entourage turned to leave Loretta's bedside, she sneered in Karen's direction, and although her voice was extremely weak, she managed to say that the day before, after the change of shift, the patients had to wait an hour and a half for a nurse to come into the room. None of the staff responded to her remark.

The chart stated that Loretta's diagnoses on admission were: "multifactorial obesity, Cushing's syndrome, stage IV malignant lymphoma in remission, bony metastasis in the spine, and migratory polyarthralgias." The day before, the researcher had heard the nurses tell Dr. Long that when they told Loretta she was not due for pain medication, she opened her purse and took some Drug P, an oral narcotic. "She's an addict, you know," Dr. Long stated. On the chart was also written, "Believe a large part of her problem may be secondary to self-overdosage of Drug D [a steroid], Drug P, and sleep medications." Loretta had been on EH II previously, and several years earlier had been admitted to the Charles Psychiatric Unit with a diagnosis of schizophrenia.

In the five months before this admission, Loretta had gained a hundred pounds, which she claimed was because of "water" imbalance as a result of the steroid therapy. When the researcher introduced herself, Loretta's first response was to take out color photos of herself before her weight gain and describe the many activities she had been involved in at earlier stages in her life. Loretta was married to a "pulmonary cripple," who was confined to a wheelchair and could visit only on rare occasions. They had no children or close relatives, and both had been cared for at home by private-duty nurses until Loretta's back pain and weakness necessitated admission.

Dr. Thomas had done Loretta's history and physical examination. His first sentence began, "This Brobdingnagian female . . . ," a phrase that one of the registered nurses used as an example to the researcher of "what a very bright young man" Dr. Thomas was. After more than a week of hospitalization, Loretta's care plan was still blank. She received radiation therapy to her spine and endured several physiologic crises during her hospitalization. Her Drug P—about two hundred tablets—had been taken away from her and locked in the narcotics box. About two months later, when she was discharged to a nursing home, her husband requested it. Much to the embarrassment of the head nurse, the drug had been taken from the narcotics box and was nowhere to be found.

Dr. Long was given to playing games, such as one that the staff called, "Anything You Can Do I Can Do, Too." (Nurses, however, played along.) Dr. Fisher had overcome his earlier bias against having nurses give standard intravenous chemotherapy and had started having Midge, the nurse employed in his office who had been a head nurse of EH II, come on rounds three times a week to do this. Dr. Long had had a similar plan at one time, but the nurse was no longer employed by him. One afternoon, while rounds were in progress, the telephone rang for the head nurse. When she returned to the group, she pleasantly announced that Mrs. Carr, the daughter of Mrs. Luckman, who had died on the unit, had been approved as a volunteer and had been assigned to EH II one-half day a week, as she had requested.

Immediately, Dr. Long said, "I'd like my [fourteen-year-old] daughter to come in on weekends and take care of my patients."

The supervisor said, "You mean she'd like to be a Candy Striper?" (Candy Stripers are high school students who undergo brief formal training for minor volunteer work.)

"No," said Dr. Long, "I don't want her to be one of those volunteer ladies who potsy around here with nothing better to do. I want her to actually take care of my patients. That's no different than a nurse coming in to do chemotherapy."

The supervisor attempted to clarify by asking, "You mean bathe them and things like that?"

Dr. Long replied, "Yes, like a nurse's aide. She's good. She works for me in the office."

When the supervisor realized he was serious, she said, "Well, I'll have to check with Mrs. Bowman [the Director of Nursing] about that." Dr. Long pursued this request until it was denied because of his daughter's lack of qualifications, including her age, for an aide's position.

The Charles School of Nursing students could be readily identified by their colored uniforms. Many of them worked part time in the hospital as aides and wore a standard white uniform. The students said that doctors treated them with more respect and afforded them a different status in the work situation when they did not realize they were nursing students. One student, a few weeks before her graduation, added:

> Doctors like to tell students things, but they don't like to listen to them. They don't like you to tell them things. When I'm in ICU working and they don't recognize I'm a student, then they listen. Today I told Dr. Fisher something about Mrs. Emmett. I was in the room with her all morning, and the head nurse wasn't in there at all. He asked her, "Is that right?"
>
> Student nurses aren't people. They make you feel like, "What am I doing here at all?" Senior nursing student—immediate idiot. I'm going to be so happy when I get out of school.

A hospital policy stated that doctors were supposed to use only one chart at a time rather than take all their patients' charts from the rack. This policy originated in territorial disputes on teaching units, that is, units with a large number of medical students, interns, and residents. But the policy was not enforced on the Oncology Unit, even though it was sometimes inconvenient for nurses who wanted to chart or students who had to leave for class. One day Dr. Fisher, the medical director of the unit, had all his charts in the conference room. A senior nursing student (described by her instructor as being "rather casual") in her last clinical experience before graduation, went in and took a chart she needed that the doctor wasn't using.

He frowned, and she said, "My, we're in a good mood this morning." He called her back and spoke to her about being rude. She told her instructor she had been "trying to get him in a better mood." The next day the instructor said the doctor "jumped on" the students for their charting, stating their notes were too long. The instructor was at the nurses' station later, quite angry, and said:

> The doctors are self-centered and egotistical, particularly with reference to their objections over integrated progress notes. They don't understand that progress notes aren't for them. It's the patient's record, not the doctor's. And the nurses cater to the doctors. The head nurse tried to oblige the doctors by having the students indent their notes from the margin. My observation was that the students' notes gave better information about the patients than any of the staff's.

Nurses did not like to have the doctors question them in front of patients. The supervisor said they particularly objected to Dr. Long's way of asking about obscure medical conditions and added: "They've told him about it, but he still does it. If he asked another doctor, he wouldn't know the answer. The nurses know the type of person he is, but they don't quite know how to deal with him."

The researcher observed a situation in which a patient described some symptoms to Dr. Long. He looked at Annette, Mildred, and one of the LPNs and asked: "What's his diagnosis?" The nurses started guessing. When they didn't give the correct answer, he asked: "How do you know the difference between radiation esophagitis and drug-induced esophagitis?" Nobody answered. "It's like a burn," Dr. Long told them, "you wait for it to ease off." As the patient looked on, Dr. Long wrote an order for viscous Xylocaine to be kept at the bedside for the patient to take as needed.

In another situation, a group went to see twenty-three-year-old Tommy Davis, a clinic patient who had leukemia. To isolate him somewhat from exposure to infection, one bed had been removed from a two-bed room. Tommy was receiving an investigational chemotherapy protocol and was also receiving an antibiotic, neomycin, which decreases the normal bacteria count in the colon, thus decreasing the chance of secondary infection. Dr. Thomas asked the nurses on rounds with him, "Why is Tommy getting the neomycin?" When nobody answered, Dr.

Thomas said, "I guess I'm talking to the air." He then explained the purpose of the drug and said to the patient, who very much wanted to go home:

> So you see, Tommy, that a lot of secondary infections arise from organisms normally present in the bowel. If I send you out, your count is so decreased that you could get a disastrous infection. That happened to me once. I let a patient go home and within two days he had a 105° temperature and died.

Tommy, who customarily spoke very little, nodded as usual, but didn't speak. Then the doctor asked, "How's your rear end today?" (Tommy also had hemorrhoids.)

Deference

Standing mute on rounds without contributing significant nursing information about patients in a systematic way was one way nurses deferred to the doctors. Occasionally, a nurse would speak up. For example, when the group went with Dr. Long to see Mrs. Juan, Dr. Long sat on the bed and auscultated her chest through her gown and robe. He commented that she looked as if she was losing weight. "Get a gallium scan," he said to the head nurse, who replied, "The prep for that is terrible—pills by mouth; she's already complaining of nausea." Dr. Long said, "Then get an indium scan. That's IV."

Deference to doctors was also shown in the ways that different individuals were addressed. Doctors referred to nurses collectively as "the girls," and individually by first name. (The supervisor and head nurse also referred to the nursing staff as the girls.) Nursing staff addressed the doctors by title only. The success of secondary socialization to status differences between nurses and doctors was illustrated by Mildred, who had graduated from a generic baccalaureate program some twenty years previously. Mildred was a neighbor of Dr. Thomas's and he told her to call him by his first name in social situations. "I could never do that," Mildred told the researcher.

Dr. Thomas appeared willing to break down traditional barriers in other ways, but the nurses were not. One day the researcher accompanied him and the head nurse to the cafeteria for lunch. It was very crowded and difficult to see three empty seats. Dr. Thomas, who got through the line first, noted that the adjacent doctors' dining room had many vacant tables, so he asked Karen, "Can you eat in the doctors' dining room?" She shook her head negatively. He then located three seats wedged against the dividing rail of the cashier's line.

Dr. Thomas' coversations with the nursing staff were also less formal. For example, one day the following dialogue took place at the nurses' station between Dr. Thomas and an LPN.

"My nurse decided she isn't making enough money so she's looking for another job," said Dr. Thomas.

"Why don't you pay her more?" asked Ruth.

"Why don't you stick your head in a toilet someplace?" retorted Dr. Thomas.

An RN interrupted and said, "I know a nurse who was working for a doctor [Long] who's looking for a job."

"I don't want any tainted nurses. I don't want anyone upon whom the black curse has been put," replied Dr. Thomas.

The nurses were laughing one day because Dr. Thomas arrived at the nurses' station when Dr. Fisher was there. Dr. Thomas flaunted convention by greeting the nurses but ignoring the chief of the unit. With the three doctors not on speaking terms, the head nurse said, "Can you imagine what it would be like if all three doctors showed up for rounds at the same time?"

The supervisor and the head nurse frequently bemoaned the fact that Dr. Long always came on the unit with an issue or a challenge. One day he brought along a "physician's assistant" to do the admission histories and physicals on his patients. The supervisor questioned this, since physician's assistants at that time were not licensed in the state. When Dr. Long told her that he had permission from Dr. Jones, the hospital administrator, she believed him. Further follow-up, however, revealed that Dr. Jones had denied Dr. Long's request to use a physician's assistant to do histories and physicals, because of the state regulation. A copy of Dr. Jones' letter of denial was given to the supervisor. That day when she arrived on the unit, the researcher was warned, "Dr. Long is not in a good mood. He found out he can't use a physician's assistant."

While the nursing staff was unanimous in their respect for the manner in which Dr. Fisher treated his patients, they sometimes had problems dealing with him. The supervisor said:

> We all handle the strain in a different way. Dr. Fisher gets mood swings and when he's down, everything is lousy; nothing is right. He'll go like that for two to three weeks. Karen was really upset the first time, because she hadn't seen him like that before. It has to take its toll on everyone who works here.

In time, the nurses identified Dr. Fisher's low moods as having a cycle of about five weeks. They'd laugh and say, "Dr. Fisher's having his period again." They recognized the legitimacy of some of his complaints, but they resented some of the way he dealt with the staff.

Several times the researcher had heard Dr. Fisher complain about the management of pain. When she asked him about it, he said, "Pain management is a chronic problem on the unit; not on days, sometimes on three-to-eleven, and always on eleven-to-seven when the regular nurse [a part-timer] is off. Certain things are not done."

One morning the researcher observed Dr. Fisher arrive on the unit. He was annoyed because the family of one of his patients had called him during the night and said Mr. Carter was in pain. Annette, who was in charge of the unit that day, started to make rounds with him. Outside Mr. Carter's room he said to her, "Unless these people are given their medication for pain as it is ordered for them, we are defeating the purpose of this unit. I have asked the nurses repeatedly to call me if a patient needs pain relief. Why don't they call?"

Annette answered, "Well, it is wrong, but maybe the reason is that not all doctors are alike, and at times the nurses have been yelled at because they called the other doctors."

"Well, they're not me," siad Dr. Fisher sternly, "and I don't know what I have to do to get the message across."

"I'll spread the word," responded Annette.

On another occasion Dr. Fisher complained to the charge nurse about patients not getting their pain medication. "There's no reason for it. The nurses know they can call me if they have any questions about a patient's pain medication. It defeats the purpose of the unit if patients have to bargain or beg for their medication."

Annette was provoked by another situation. A patient had had diarrhea all night, and the family called Dr. Fisher. The researcher was told that when he and Annette got to the patient's bedside, Dr. Fisher "yelled" at Annette because the patient hadn't received any medication. Later, at one of Ted's rap conferences, Annette said, "I resent being the target of his anger when I wasn't even there, and I don't like being put down in front of a patient."

Ted said, "It's part of the pecking order that the buck is passed downward."

Nurses rarely confronted doctors with what they regarded as unjust criticism, nor did there seem to be a coordinated effort through all three shifts to resolve the recurrent problem of pain management through a staff education program. Dr. Fisher said he attempted to deal with the problem by putting certain patients on regularly scheduled medication rather than p.r.n. (as needed), which required a patient's request or a nursing judgment.

However, the head nurse said that Dr. Fisher wrote "strange" pain medication orders. "He'll order one thing, and then he'll write, give another thing if the first is ineffective, and then a third thing, if the other two don't work." This meant that a lot of orders he wrote had to be clarified directly with him. He also wanted some patients awakened at night to keep them on a regular pain medication schedule, while others he didn't want awakened.

The researcher asked if Dr. Fisher was told that he was writing confusing orders. The head nurse responded:

He's forgetful; he'll write something on the progress notes that he plans to do, then forget to write it on the order sheet. I'll gently remind him that he didn't order. Like I'll say, "Were you planning on doing such and such a thing?" He says he's always accessible, but he isn't. One day he told me to call him in an hour if a patient didn't get pain relief. I tried for three hours before I finally reached him.

One day Dr. Fisher wrote an order for "B-12 monthly." Karen went after him to ask how much. He said, "1,000 micrograms." She then asked him if he really meant monthly, and he replied affirmatively. Since the patient was almost ready for discharge and orders had to be rewritten every seven days, the significance of this order was questionable. When Karen got back to the desk she picked up the chart of another patient of Dr. Fisher's and said, "Oh, he didn't renew those meds. He's so naughty. I'm going to take this right back to him."

One week in November, the researcher observed that Karen, who was generally placid and pleasant, appeared quite dejected. The researcher inquired about her observation. Karen explained that a few days previously, Dr. Fisher told her in the morning that he was going to try to call in Mr. Santiago for readmission. Since there were three other patients on the call-in list, Dr. Fisher agreed to call her before three-thirty so she would know whether to call in another patient. Karen explained that it had turned out to be a very bad day; Annette went home sick, and Lisa didn't feel well. There were a number of crises that had to be dealt with. At four-thirty, when Karen was finally ready to leave, ten hours after her arrival, she hadn't heard from Dr. Fisher's office about Mr. Santiago, so she called in another patient.

The next morning on rounds, Dr. Fisher told Karen that he hadn't been able to get in touch with Mr. Santiago. Karen mistakenly said, "That's good, because I called in someone else when I didn't hear from you."

"You did what? I would have thought you would have had the consideration to call me before you went home," was Karen's recall of Dr. Fisher's indignant response.

She continued:

Believe me, with the day I had, that's the last thing I would have thought of. Then he wrote on the chart that he had ordered electrolytes on a patient yesterday and "please do them today." But I had called him on the phone yesterday and given him the results. I was going to confront him with it because he really hurt my feelings, because I go out of my way to do things for him. I call him on things that are really his responsibility.

Karen went on to say that Dr. Fisher's manner was the same on the other hospital units, and the consensus was that he was probably having family problems. After talking the situation over with her husband,

Karen decided not to confront Dr. Fisher because "I'd just bringing myself down to his level. I really was hurt about it, but I just let it ride." Karen explained that she was pleasant to him while he was on the unit but didn't offer any extra conversation. At the end of the week he resumed his usual manner, offering a friendly, "Hi, Karen," as if nothing had ever happened.

Since there was no regular intern or resident assigned to EH II, nurses had to call the attending physicians directly, which involved some trepidation. As Lisa said, "With Dr. Long, you're damned if you do, and you're damned if you don't. Sometimes when you call he asks you why bother him with such trivia, and sometimes for similar circumstances he asks why wasn't he called."

One night, after the eleven o'clock report, the researcher heard Ellen, the evening-shift graduate nurse, tell Catherine, the oncoming night nurse, that Mr. Kravitz had fallen, cutting his neck and bending his glasses. Ellen said, "The resident saw him, but I didn't call Dr. Long. Should I have?"

Catherine shrugged and said that one night at her request the resident called him a second time about Mrs. Wales. "I got on the phone and Long asked me why I was calling him twice. I told him because she's your patient."

Mrs. Wales had been admitted during the evening from the emergency room and Dr. Long had come in to see her about eleven. After he left, medical residents were in charge of her treatment. She had been discharged from the Oncology Unit a few months earlier after radiation treatment of pelvic metastases. Her X-ray studies at that time showed a tumor impinging on her ureters.

Dr. Long had been seeing Mrs. Wales in his office. She lived alone and apparently had been in failing health for only a few days following her last office visit. This time she was admitted with kidney failure. Her adult children, who brought her to the hospital, said that she did not want them to visit her and that they had not talked to her in two days. Mrs. Wales had had a colostomy for some time following surgery for cancer of the colon. The nurses recalled that she took care of her colostomy but didn't have to irrigate often. When she did an irrigation, however, she was so conscious of privacy that she locked herself in the bathroom and wouldn't let anyone in until she had finished.

This time, when the semicomatose Mrs. Wales was put into bed and the nurses were undressing her, they noticed that her underpants were lined with stacks of paper towels, which she had apparently used in a vain attempt to absorb the foul-smelling, bloody discharge from the colostomy. As the nurses were attempting to peel off the towels and clean her, the odor was so bad that Pat, the charge nurse, had to leave the room twice to vomit. When the nurses got the drainage cleaned off Mrs.

Wales's skin, they noted that she was covered with "septic hives," or large abscesses.

Ellen asked the family members why they hadn't cleaned her before bringing her to the hospital. They replied that they just wanted to get her help as quickly as possible. Ellen also asked the emergency room supervisor why they hadn't done anything for Mrs. Wales since she had been held there for a few hours. The supervisor showed Ellen a list of eighteen patients with greater immediate needs.

Mrs. Wales lived until noon the next day. During that time, the residents made three unsuccessful attempts to reestablish urinary flow with drugs. These attempts were upsetting to Vicki, the young registered nurse assigned to Mrs. Wales on the day shift. Vicki believed the patient was aware that the residents were "working on her," though she was unable to speak, and she thought Mrs. Wales should have been made comfortable and permitted to die peacefully.

Despite the problematic situations described, it was the nursing staff's consensus that physician-nurse relationships on the Oncology Unit were better than those in other parts of Charles Hospital. The researcher asked Lisa, who had graduated from the Charles School one and one-half years previously, if she thought the model of physician-nurse relationships was hierarchical or interdependent. She replied:

> Well, it fluctuates a bit. There's times when the doctor freaks out and he's God and we are supposed to do what he says. That's mostly in the rest of the hospital. Here, sometimes they say why don't you do things for yourself. Use your own head. We can interrelate or blend our roles or whatever. There are times when they ask us for our opinion. I think Dr. Fisher is a little more of the traditional model. He puts himself at the top, but he's smart enough to ask us and to deal with us the way he knows he should, although he really has the attitude that he's the head man. Long is like that, too.

Lisa stated that the quality of nurse-physician relationships also had to do with the way the nurse presents herself. "If she presents herself in a subservient way, that's the role she'll play."

The researcher asked Lisa how she was socialized in her Charles nursing school experience. She replied:

> In between. We had a lot of instructors who were around Charles Hospital for a long time. So doctors were gods in a lot of ways, and everything was oriented to them. Then we got some younger instructors who told us you don't have to do everything a doctor says just because he says it. You have to think for yourself and develop working relationships.

Doctors' Coping Mechanisms

The researcher asked the doctors how they coped with the unending tragedies and crises associated with the daily treatment of patients with cancer. Dr. Thomas told the researcher, "You get into these things by default. Hematology is my diversion. I guess I have my own defense mechanism."

Dr. Fisher stressed that he had a strong family life but added:

I do get depressed at times. A series of patient crises would cause this. But there is no more problem with depression than orthopedists or neurologists have with their type of patients. No more, just different. Cancer is looked upon as different by the culture.

Dr. Long replied: "I get high—manic. I use humor. In the office I spend more time telling jokes than talking about the patient's illness. They need that."

On another occasion, Dr. Long, looking somber after saying that two of his patients had died on another unit within two minutes of each other, said, "It's hard. You care for these patients and they become your friends, and then you lose them."

REFERENCES

1. Dunphy, J. E. Annual discourse—on caring for the patient with cancer. *N. E. J. Med.*, 295: 318, 1976.

Chapter 5
The Nursing Staff

This chapter is concerned with members of the nursing staff, defined here as including the supervisor, head nurse, staff registered nurses (RNs), licensed practical nurses (LPNs), a technician, and aides. A ward clerk was assigned to the unit. Data presented were collected primarily, though not exclusively, on the day shift. Aspects of staffing, work organization and performance, professional ideology-reality conflicts, role discrepancies, work stresses, and collective and individual coping mechanisms are addressed.

NURSING STAFF MEMBERS

When data collection started, the day staff were:

Frances Kiely	RN, Supervisor	Full time
Karen Foster	RN, Head Nurse	Full time
Lisa Gerardi	RN, Staff Nurse	Full time
Annette Beck	RN, BSN, Staff Nurse	Full time
Mildred Hayes	RN, BSN, Staff Nurse	Part time (4 days)
Libby MacGregor	RN, Staff Nurse	Part time (3 days)
June Horvath	RN, A.S., Staff Nurse	Part time (2 days)
Ruth Veston	LPN	Full time
Sharon Funesti	LPN	Full time
Marlene Rush	LPN	Full time
Vivian Nichols	LPN	Full time
Julie Beltran	Technician	Full time
Alice Boardman	Aide	Full time
Dolly Henry	Ward Clerk	Full time

There was some rotation of day staff RNs to the evening shift, but this was minimal.

About one month later, at the end of June, the following staff were employed to complete the unit:

Donna Carro	GN*, BSN	Full time
Ellen Metzger	GN, diploma	Full time
Jill Wells	Aide, BA	Full time

Though the unit now had its full complement of staff, this number did not provide for additional staff coverage for vacations, holidays, weekends, personal illness, or staff crises, or evening-shift coverage for vacation or other staff absence. These exigencies depleted the actual work force.

The evening staff members were:

Patricia Harris	RN	Full time
Sara Hamilton	RN	Part time
Clare Nelson	LPN	Full time
Rosa Mercolo	LPN	Full time
Adele Furmer	Aide	Full time
Brenda Post	Aide	Full time

Since the night-staff schedule was made out by the night supervisor and posted only in the nursing office, neither day staff nor patients knew in advance which RNs or LPNs would be assigned to the Oncology Unit on any particular night. The researcher met the following night-shift members:

Catherine Green	RN	Part time
Paula Lynn	RN	Part time
Toni Campbell	RN	Part time
Ed Toth	LPN	Full time
Mabel Jones	LPN	Part time
Carrie Nolan	Aide	Full time

The Day Staff

Supervisor. Frances Kiely had graduated from the hospital school about thirty years earlier. She had been promoted to supervisor after experience as a head nurse at Charles. She opened EH II as a Self-Care Unit and remained its supervisor when it became the Oncology Unit. She was also the supervisor of the Psychiatric Unit and the Self-Care Unit,

---

* The classification GN (Graduate Nurse) refers to new graduates who were scheduled to take the state registered nurse license examination shortly after they started their first job. They were not permitted to perform the full role functions of RNs; for example, GNs could not give intravenous heparin.

EH I. She worked the day shift but took her turn on weekends "covering the house," that is, being responsible for supervision of all nursing units. At the end of the research year she received a baccalaureate degree in health care administration from a state college.

The supervisor had administrative responsibility for patients, nurses, and physical facilities of the three units. She said of the Oncology Unit:

> Staff turnover is about what it is on other units. No one left because they were dissatisfied with the unit, oncology, or interpersonal relations. Karen Foster is the fourth head nurse. Two of the others got married and moved away and one retired. We got rid of one aide who caused constant disruption. We try to be open, and I really feel we would know of staff problems. You like to think that they say what they think to me. I think they do.

The staff appeared to like and be at ease with Mrs. Kiely, who had a quiet, casual manner. One LPN said:

> I can relate better to my supervisor than to the head nurse. I know her better. We started this floor together. She's available to me anytime. I can talk to her better than Karen. There's been four head nurses on this floor since it started, but only one supervisor.

On the other hand, a registered nurse, when speaking about a patient, Jim Jason, stated, "If only my supervisor were more alert, we could present this case [publish it in a nursing journal]. He was the most difficult situation we have ever had on this floor. I hold it against someone who is not progressive."

Head nurse. Karen Foster had graduated from a hospital school about twenty years earlier and after her marriage she left active nursing for twelve years. The youngest of her three sons was presently a teenager. Karen had returned to nursing at Charles two years previously, working two nights a week in the Intensive Care Unit, after her husband became unemployed. When the researcher asked if that wasn't a difficult place to start after being away for twelve years, Karen replied, "In the Intensive Care Unit you sink or swim, and I swam."

When she heard of the opening for a head nurse on EH II, a year before this research started, she applied for and got the job. She attended a part-time four-week management course given for head nurses by the Inservice Education Department. Thus, though a willing learner, Karen was a relative newcomer to the role of head nurse and the specialty of oncology nursing. During the research year she completed courses at an off-campus site of a state college and graduated with a baccalaureate degree in health care administration. (As a personnel benefit, full-time nurses at Charles were reimbursed $200 per year for matriculated college study; part-time nurses were allowed $100.) Both Karen and Frances, the supervisor, expressed resentment to the researcher that the state university's College of Nursing, located on its Lafayette campus, "does nothing for the RN."

The head nurse, who had a calm, positive, and realistic manner with a quiet sense of humor, set the tone for the unit. She was concerned about patients, families, and her staff. She was recognized as the leader by the nursing staff, and she had the respect of the physicians and the support of the supervisor.

Karen's manner was casual and pleasant, but reserved. Her facial expression didn't change much in response to many types of adverse situations. After particularly stressful periods, she was subject to migraine headaches and/or dermatitis on her hands. Karen said she "loved" her work on the Oncology Unit, adding philosophically, "There is a master plan; if my husband hadn't been laid off, I'd still be making peanut butter and jelly sandwiches."

By virtue of her recent experience in the Intensive Care Unit, Karen was also the most technically skilled nurse on the unit. When Jim Jason returned to EH II from the ICU on a stretcher with a myriad of tubes, pumps, IVs, and dressings, Karen left her role as "acting ward clerk," accompanied him to his room, and directed the staff nurses in his immediate care. When four IV-team members failed to accomplish a venipuncture for Mr. Henry to receive a blood transfusion, Karen was asked to do it and was immediately successful. She explained or demonstrated to the staff the use of the infusion pump for chemotherapy via the hepatic artery. Although, according to the nursing department's expectations, the head nurse decentralized her authority by using four team leaders and four teams to deliver patient care, the staff frequently bypassed the leaders and sought technical information or direction directly from her.

Staff registered nurses. These were graduates of either hospital diploma schools, associate degree programs, or generic baccalaureate nursing programs. They were licensed to practice in the state, although some had received their initial licensure in other states. They were expected to perform all levels of nursing care required by patients and to be team leaders. The full-time registered nurses were expected, after an "orientation to the desk," to take charge of the unit in the head nurse's absence.

Mildred Hayes had graduated with a BSN from a five-year program twenty years previously. She dropped out of nursing for sixteen years, but after a traumatic divorce she sought work and considered herself lucky to get a job at Charles, since she had never worked in a hospital. When she had come to Charles, three years previously, Mildred said she was told by the then-new director of nursing, "I'll put you on a self-care cancer floor where you can learn at your own rate."

Mildred added:

They were starting their first nurse refresher course then, but she refused to put me in it because she thought I'd be bored. The way I had to learn and adjust to the floor was very unfair. Within six weeks I had to run the floor, and they didn't have the baby-sitting program to orient you to the floor like they do now.

When I started, every other weekend there was one nurse in charge and on meds for the floor and no clerk. I put in a year like that, and it was pure hell. I worked from 6:20 A.M. to 4:30 P.M. without a bite to eat. A year ago Dr. Fisher did put in for overtime for us. I can't leave until I know things are done.

Mildred was actively looking for a new job and had gone from full time to four days a week as the research started.

Annette Beck had worked as an aide on EH II during summer vacations from the state university's nursing program. She received a baccalaureate degree and had been employed on the unit for about a year when the research began. She chose EH II because she liked the staff and thought the nursing care was good.

Donna Carro had also worked at Charles during summer vacations from her baccalaureate nursing program at a private university. As a "floating aide," she had had the chance to observe many units; she chose to work on EH II, because, "I saw good nursing care practiced there." Donna left Charles Hospital after six months. After her initial "honeymoon" period of orientation and functioning as a team member, she was unable to make the necessary adaptation to the continuing stresses of patients' conditions (particularly dying patients) and the increased role-performance expectations of her employer.

When the study started Lisa Gerard had been working on the unit for about a year after her graduation from Charles School of Nursing. Her first choice of work was on the Psychiatric Unit, but there were no vacancies. Oncology was her second choice because, "I felt I could get good experience in psychiatry, which I love, and medicine, which I like."

Libby MacGregor, a sixty-nine-year-old, physically fit RN, worked three days a week. She had graduated from a hospital school in 1933 and dropped out of nursing for twenty-three years after her marriage. She told the researcher that four years previously she had fractured her ankle while working on another ward, and "after I came back they put me here. I wasn't very happy about it at first, but I've gotten use to it. I liked surgical floors—most surgical patients recover and go home." Libby was to retire in March, but she again applied for and received a one-year extension. She said:

I'm the grandmother of the unit. I'm twice as old as the others. I don't mind the work, though I'm tired when I get home; but I recuperate. I grew up on a farm, and I always had had work to do. . . . They don't know what a good hard day's work is, some of these kids.

When talking with the researcher about dying patients, Libby commented, "Death used to bother me more forty years ago than it does now. These younger ones get so emotional about it. Why I never cried when my father died." As Libby described the last days of her father's life, the tears came to her eyes, and she added, "Maybe that's why I'm crying now."

June Horvath was an LPN who went on to receive an associate degree in nursing from a community college and RN licensure. She worked three days a week "to keep active." She was assigned to the Oncology Unit because there was no other opening when she wanted to start work.

Ellen Metzger started working in June after graduation from a hospital school. She was oriented on days but was hired for the three-to-eleven shift. There were no openings on other units. Ellen worked on the unit for about eight months, then after failing her state licensing exam for the second time, she transferred to another unit as an aide. The supervisor said:

> She didn't work out there either. She continued to come in late. Her boyfriend was the cause of a lot of her difficulty. She was supporting him, and she owned the car. The staff would see her with him in the parking garage when she was supposed to be up here getting report. Many evenings she'd come in upset after a fight with him—once they were arguing on the way to work, and he rear-ended another car. I told her to go home when she called in, but she didn't. The evening supervisor spent a good deal of time getting her examined in the emergency room and getting a tranquilizer to calm her down.

Vicki Martin, a graduate from another hospital school in Lafayette, arrived in mid-December. She wanted a day job with little shift rotation. Her social life was a high priority. At the end of the research year, Vicki was described as "still flaky," implying that she paid little attention to details and had low commitment to cancer patients.

Rita Reyes, in her late thirties, arrived in early spring. New to the region, she was a recent associate-degree graduate from a distant area of the country. She wanted part-time work three days a week, and the Oncology Unit had the only opening. Rita had considerable difficulty adjusting to the unit but remained because she could not get the hours she wanted on another unit. Rita commented:

> In the state I come from they are much more strict, and nurses are much more accountable. We had to chart every two hours—things are lax here. I'm very disappointed in the nursing aspects. Here the emphasis is on procedures and vital signs. They are chronically short of supplies, including IV tubing and fluids. Where I come from they are better supplied—patient comfort comes first. There is no clinical orientation at all here.
>
> I like the staff—that's the reason I've stayed here.

Mary Manfreda also came in the spring for two days a week, and

Louise Jackson came full time in May after having taken a nurse refresher course in a nearby hospital. Mary and Louise were returning to nursing after drop-out periods from nursing of twelve and eighteen years, respectively.

Licensed practical nurses. These were graduates of a one-year program who had passed the state licensing exam. They were prepared to work under the supervision of registered nurses. There were four full-time LPNs on the day shift, two on the evening shift, and one on the night shift. Working days, Ruth Veston, Marlene Rush, and Sharon Funesti, all in their thirties, were first-year graduates of the county's vocational education program. Because of hypertension and job and family pressures, Ruth went from full time to four days a week in December.

Vivian Nichols had graduated about ten years previously from an eighteen-month program in the South. As the study year ended, Vivian went from full time to a four-day week also.

Technician. This was an unlicensed position with a scope of practice "somewhere between an aide and an LPN." Julie, the technician on the Oncology Unit, had been a registered nurse in her own country, the Philippines, but did not pass the licensing examinations in this country, which she attributed to difficulties in reading and writing English. She had been on the unit for about four years. She wept as she spoke of her lost status:

> I can do treatments but not medicines and injections or IVs. I'm an RN in my own country. Sometimes (here) I'm in the situation where I know more. I feel it not for me but because of the patient. If you were in their place would you like to have a thermometer put back in your mouth dirty? Mucus dries and is hardened. I wipe it off with alcohol and rinse it first. [Weeping] I think it is my pride. I have a feeling that I can't do a thing. I have that feeling of being dumb. I am put down. The only consolation I have is that in my category of work I am very close to the patient. I don't have very much hardship except when I take care of patients who are like dying. I get attached, and I get the depression, I shed tears, but I still continue my nursing. I feel sad like they are my relatives.

Julie perceived that she was rejected by some patients. In describing this, she said:

> Sometimes I really cry; some yell at me. Some pretend they are sleeping. I feel that they don't like me. But maybe it is part of their sickness. Sometimes I think it is because of my color. I just take it the whole day—the next day I'll tell them [team leaders] what happened, and I won't be assigned. They are mostly men—they are really hard to handle when it comes to psychology. I never had psychology really. I'm not really good at dealing with the emotional problems patients have.

Aides. At Charles the aides generally received a short training in the hygienic and comfort care of patients and performance of some simple treatments. In the researcher's experience, the two aides on the day shift on the Oncology Unit were exceptional. Alice Boardman, a sixty-five-year-old woman who retired near the end of the study year, had a remarkable degree of physical energy and an attitude of cheerful realism with the patients. She had come to Charles eleven years previously to be an aide after her son died of Hodgkin's disease. He had been hospitalized at Charles several times, and the unmet needs of patients motivated her to seek this work.

The second aide, Jill Wells, was a twenty-three-year-old college graduate who had majored in German language and literature and had held a good-paying position in the international loan division of a prominent bank. That job did not give her sufficient satisfaction, so she enrolled in a technical school for eight weeks of accelerated aide training, which did not include patient contact. She was drawn to nursing for religious and humanitarian reasons. When she sought employment at Charles, she agreed to work on the Oncology Unit. For one day she worked with patients along with Alice Boardman and then "was on my own," with a full patient assignment as a team member. Her hospital orientation program was scheduled for one month after she started working. Jill was also taking evening college courses to meet qualifications for admission to a baccalaureate nursing program the next academic year. When asked about her unemployed husband's reaction to the salary differential between a bank loan officer and a nurses' aide ($3.60 per hour), Jill replied, "The job I had was high paying and not physically demanding at all. But I was miserable in that job, and he's pleased that I like to get up in the morning and go to my work now." (Her husband had had an unexpected job layoff.)

Ward clerk. This category of worker received on-the-job training from an experienced clerk and was assigned to a unit by a nursing supervisor. Clerks were supposed to do the secretarial and clerical tasks of unit management under the direction of the head nurse. There was no clerk assigned to EH II on weekends and only occasionally was there one on the evening shift. In a clerk's absence the head nurse or charge nurse assumed the clerk's role functions.

Volunteers. Three women volunteered their services one half day each week, helping with patient diversionary activities or distributing mail. One woman had breast cancer, one was the wife of a staff internist, and one was the daughter of a patient who had died after several admissions to EH II.

Role Boundaries

A large part of the supervisor's and head nurse's time and effort was concerned with seeing that other departments did their work. For example, in the early spring, the patient rooms were emptied one at a time and stripped for painting in light pastel shades. The staff attributed this improvement to Dr. Fisher's intercession with the new administration. When the work in one three-bed room seemed about to be completed, the head nurse called in three patients. However, the beds could not be put back until the baseboards were painted and the Maintenance Department stripped and waxed the floors. The maintenance man arrived before the painters and started to wax the floor without stripping it, so the painter was delayed until the wax dried. The Housekeeping Department wouldn't replace the metal covers on the overhead heating ducts because their department was supposed to handle them only if they remained in place. Since Maintenance unscrewed them for painting, Maintenance would have to screw them back. Between calls to incoming patients and to Housekeeping and Maintenance, the head nurse answered Dr. Long's questions about patients, drew up a syringe full of Adriamycin for him to give a patient, looked up a drug in the *Physician's Desk Reference,* and called the pharmacy for additional information. Over a four-hour period the supervisor and head nurse spent large intervals trying to get the room in order. "If we did everything ourselves, we would have been done hours ago," said Karen.

When all the rooms on EH II were painted, Maintenance started peeling the loose vinyl covering off the corridor walls, but then decided it was Housekeeping's job to clean the walls for painting. The walls remained a partially peeled mess for over a month. After unsuccessful attempts to mediate the dispute, the supervisor wrote to the vice-president of operations, requesting that he settle the boundary dispute and have the walls painted.

Professional boundaries were problematic also. For example, after an unannounced inspection by the state health department, Dr. Jones, the president, and Mrs. Bowman, vice-president and director of nursing services, issued the following memo to the nursing staff:

> Comments re. deficiencies found at unannounced state licensure inspection conducted on January 11 and 12:
>
> Nursing staff may not accept or carry out unsigned or incomplete orders.
>
> No verbal orders are to be carried out after 18 hours.
>
> All specific time limits must be rigorously adhered to by nursing staff.
>
> Unlicensed physicians' orders must be countersigned.

The researcher commented to the supervisor that the directives concerned nurses monitoring doctors doing their jobs, or having to bear the consequences of patient complaints or inadequacies in patient treatment. The supervisor commented, "Naturally. Not only that, there were three different memos issued in three days on the same subject, one canceling out the other. We're also supposed to see that doctors date their histories and physicals, too."

Once the researcher saw the supervisor in the first floor hallway. She was going to the Xerox machine to copy a few pages of progress notes from the chart of one of the Psychiatric Unit patients. The doctor had gone on vacation and had written several days progress notes in advance, including a discharge note.

The researcher asked a key informant about the head nurse's over-involvement in the work of other departments, and the professional employee commented, "Head nurses being middle management is new. They don't realize what their rights are. Most head nurses are three-year graduates going for degrees in nonnursing majors."

"What do you think will change this situation here?" the researcher asked.

"Young head nurses won't tolerate this. They are hearing more on women's rights. It's much better for them to speak up."

Staffing Crisis

A series of critical events on the unit, combined with Karen's personal crises, made the last months of the year and the first half of the next year a particularly stressful time for the staff. These events included not having a ward clerk; two experienced RNs, Annette and Lisa, resigning with no full-time replacements; having no full-time RNs prepared to take charge of the unit in the head nurse's absence; adaptational crisis of a new staff RN; and attempting to have part-timers replace full-time RNs.

In October, Dolly Henry, who was said to be a good ward clerk when she was present, was fired for too-frequent absenteeism. Although this was to have a critical effect on the head nurse's work, the staff's initial response was positive. A group discussing the situation agreed that it was good that Charles "finally had the courage to fire someone," rather than continuing to tolerate irresponsible or undependable behavior.

Unfortunately, no clerk was available to replace Dolly, and this situation continued for more than four months. The head nurse or, in her absence the charge nurse, took over the duties of the ward clerk for this period. Although the nurses resented this situation and made their views known to the nursing supervisor, who agreed with them, they did not protest to the hospital administrator responsible for ward clerks. The supervisor was told there were no qualified applicants. One of the ward clerk's duties was to stamp an addressograph plate on every page of a patient's chart and on requests to the laboratory, X-Ray, or other departments. Three addressographed stick-on labels had to accompany each specimen as well as the addressographed request slip. One day at four-thirty the head nurse was still at the desk taking orders off a newly admitted patient's chart. A "float" ward clerk was at the addressograph making labels. The nursing supervisor in charge of ward clerks came by and told the clerk to report to another unit, saying to Karen, "You don't want her; she's not too sharp." Karen said nothing, but started to addressograph seventeen sets of three labels for each of the tests the doctor had ordered for the patient.

Mildred Hayes, who for a number of years had been in charge of the unit on the head nurse's days off, went from full time to four days a week. Since part-timers were not supposed to be in charge, Annette and Lisa were the only RNs able to assume charge nurse responsibilities. But in September, Lisa and Annette announced their resignations, which were not unanticipated. Lisa had planned to work for about eighteen months and then travel to another part of the country for new experiences. Annette, who had also worked on the unit about eighteen months, told the researcher:

> During my student days I had a desire to go into teaching, but I knew I needed experience. There was a poistion open in the Inservice Education Department, so I applied and I got it. I'll miss the floor, but I have a need to grow and educate myself in other areas. If I had to tell anyone a place to get experience, I'd tell them here.

Lisa left in early November without a replacement being hired. Annette had to wait to transfer to the Inservice Education Department until a replacement was hired for her. When Florence Helvas arrived in November for a three-week orientation, Annette left. Florence had worked nights for many years in another hospital in Lafayette but wanted a day position. During her three-week orientation she was gradually assigned to all nursing responsibilities on the unit, including the desk. The head nurse said, "It's such a pleasure not to have to spoon-feed somebody. She's mature and competent." But Florence resigned after three weeks; her letter of resignation said that she had become very depressed at the change in her two-year-old child who had been left with a baby sitter. (Florence also had four teenagers.) She added:

> EH II, in my opinion, is a department where *real* nursing *is* going on, and the three weeks that I worked with you were very satisfying to me. Much as I try to liberate myself, I find my first commitment is to my family—*that* is *me*.

By early December, then, there was no back-up person who could be in charge of the unit on the head nurse's day off or in case of illness. Also in early December, Karen's forty-nine-year-old husband sustained a second acute myocardial infarction and was admitted to Charles Coronary Care Unit. He was hospitalized for about three weeks and was discharged with continuing symptomatic myocardial insufficiency. While he was in the hospital, Karen usually had lunch with him in his room when this was possible and returned in the evening to visit. Simultaneously, her recurrent urinary tract infections increased in frequency and severity. She continued to work daily. One morning, after taking report, making rounds, and taking care of immediate needs on the unit, she walked to the X-Ray Department for an intravenous pyelogram. Still fasting, she returned to EH II, where several crises deterred her plan to get her lunch bag and go to her husband's room. By one o'clock she was acutely light-headed from hunger and finally went to lunch. The studies revealed kidney pathology, requiring hospitalization for further examination under anesthesia. This news was conveyed to Karen on the unit by a telephone call from her physician.

When Karen told the staff at the desk what the doctor had said about her kidney problem, (hydronephrosis and hydroureter), Libby said, "I'd better retire before things get worse and before the unit falls apart. If there's one thing I don't want to be it's in charge of this floor."

It was easy to see why Karen looked dejected the week before Christmas—a hospitalized husband having recurrent chest pain, a son at home with infectious mononucleosis, on medical treatment herself, and no one prepared to be in charge of the unit except Mildred, a part-timer, who was not given compensatory pay when she assumed the charge nurse role. The unit was even more short-staffed than usual because of holiday time schedules, and the "unit's sickest patient ever," Jim Jason, arrived from the Intensive Care Unit, and one nurse had to be assigned solely to him.

Later that week, Mildred told the staff that Karen was to be admitted to the hospital for examination with anesthesia on the first Wednesday in January and would return to work on Saturday, taking Thursday and Friday as her days off. Mildred was to be in charge of the unit on Wednesday, Thursday, and Friday. The staff raised the question of who would be in charge on Saturday if Karen couldn't come back, since Mildred was scheduled to be off. They thought Karen wasn't giving herself enough time to recover, and someone mentioned that she could be out for quite awhile if she had to have surgery.

Libby declared she wouldn't be "stuck with the desk." Mildred said she wouldn't come in to be in charge again because she was only a part-timer. Neither Vicki nor Donna was oriented to the charge nurse role; June was going on an around the world vacation trip, and she was a part-timer anyway. Another staff nurse, who was temporarily assigned to EH II while the Self-Care Unit was closed over the holiday, said she wouldn't be in charge. There was still no ward clerk. Staff suggested that Annette be brought back temporarily from Inservice Education, but this was not done.

Mildred and Libby thought Dr. Fisher should go to the nursing office and get help. Libby said that the nursing office was unsympathetic to the unit's needs, and the hospital would rather save money than hire new nurses. The previous Saturday, staffing had been so limited that Ruth complained she didn't have enough time to complete the treatments ordered for the patients on one side. Jill, the aide, said she had to keep interrupting Ruth as she was doing the treatments to ask her for help in positioning patients and getting them in and out of bed. A Charles nursing instructor commented that the unit was so short-staffed on weekends it was a wonder that staff had time to do anything besides say hello to patients.

Karen did not return to work on Saturday because she developed a severe headache following anesthesia and was too sick to work. The nursing office called in Mildred, the part-time RN, to work on her day off. When Dr. Fisher heard that Karen was going to return to work on Sunday, informants said he telephoned Frances, the supervisor, at home and "yelled" at her, saying he did not want a sick nurse heading the floor where his patients were and that she should not have scheduled Karen to work, adding, "If that girl gets sick, it's nursing's fault." Frances told Dr. Fisher that Karen made out the time schedule and put herself down to work. Dr. Fisher called Karen at home and told her she should stay home until she felt well enough to work. The supervisor called the director of nursing at her home, who said it was the first time she'd ever heard of a doctor concerned about a nurse who was ill.

Karen worked all day Sunday, but her headache got worse and she was out sick on Monday. Mildred described the subsequent incident:

> When Dr. Fisher saw that Karen came in to work on Sunday, he got Frances up here and really blasted her. He was furious that Karen came back. He told the supervisor that she should have taken care of staffing the unit. Then he went behind closed doors in the conference room and blasted her again. Frances was terribly crushed over that. Karen should be terribly honored that Dr. Fisher came to her defense.

The researcher asked, "Was his concern over Karen or the fact that his patients were at risk with no one prepared to be in charge in Karen's absence?"

"I don't know," Mildred said, "but he called Karen a few more times at home to see how she was."

Frances said that after this incident Dr. Fisher "carried a grudge" toward her for two or three weeks. She added:

> From a supervisor's point of view, Dr. Long is easier to deal with. He'll carry on about something but when it's over, he doesn't carry a grudge. But Dr. Fisher's method of not speaking for weeks is something I find more difficult to deal with.

Karen went to see a neurologist, who said her headache was caused by a reaction to the anesthesia; the anesthesiologist said that was impossible. Her kidney condition was diagnosed as a blood-vessel defect, requiring examination with anesthesia every six months for follow-up. She said, "I'm not taking that stuff again."

In January, an obstetrics nurse was assigned to EH II while her unit was closed for remodeling. Two part-time nurses were hired in March, and a full-time nurse finally in May. This nurse had been out of nursing for eighteen years and had taken a refresher course at a neighboring hospital. The remaining two full-time vacancies were filled in June by Janet and Penny, two new graduates of the hospital nursing school. Janet came because she was a well cancer patient and believed she could give a unique kind of help to the patients on EH II, as did Penny, whose younger brother had leukemia.

DIVISION OF LABOR

Team Method

Team nursing was introduced to American hospitals about 1949 to deal with the shortage of registered nurses in hospitals during and after World War II. About this time, hospitals' use of nonprofessional nursing personnel, that is, licensed practical nurses and nurse's aides, was considerably expanded.

The objective of team nursing was to plan and implement individualized "comprehensive care" for a defined group of patients by using each team member's varied levels of knowledge and abilities. To provide "comprehensive patient care" required that team leaders have more knowledge and skill in the psychological, sociological, and cultural aspects of patient care; better ability to plan care and to write plans of care for workers to follow; and better ability to conduct daily team conferences that invited the input of all members to plan the care. The team leader was to be a baccalaureate-educated registered nurse with special preparation in leadership and managerial skills necessary for supervising professional and nonprofessional nursing staff in the delivery of patient care.

Structurally, the team method provided for decentralization of the head nurse's authority and responsibility for the work of nursing staff. This freed the head nurse to concentrate on overall supervision of the care of all patients, the development of staff, and the managerial aspects of the unit. Generally, the RNs who were most skilled in bedside nursing became the team leaders, but in the process, they became further removed from direct patient care. Much of the bedside care was assigned to less-trained, less-skilled nonprofessional workers. The team leader continued to administer medications and to take care of certain aspects of direct patient care, such as treatments that were more complex than the training of the other team members allowed.

The team method was thus a departure in structure and function from the two traditional methods of nurse assignment: the functional method, in which certain levels of personnel were assigned tasks, such as distribution of medications or treatments, for all the patients on the unit; and the "case method," in which assignments were made by matching the skill level of personnel with the total tasks necessary to a patient's care, that is, patients with complex nursing needs were assigned to RNs, and those with simple care needs to aides.

Team nursing on EH II. The staff did not indicate that they were knowledgeable about the principles of team nursing, nor were these applied in practice. "Team," to the researcher, simply referred to a group of personnel assigned to care for a group of patients. A team consisted of an RN or LPN as team leader and one or more RNs, LPNs or aides as team members. There were four teams on the day shift and two on the evening and night shifts, one for each end of the "L." The day shift teams each had from five to seven patients.

Distribution of Work

Each day after the morning report, the head nurse posted the names of team leaders and members and the patients assigned to each team on the bulletin board behind the nurse's station. She attempted to distribute the patient-care load evenly among the four teams and to keep teams and patients together for one week. The patients were assigned geographically, however, to reduce the distance staff walked between rooms.

The team leader assigned patients and/or tasks for herself and her team members. Team leaders generally gave the medications and injections and supervised the intravenous therapy, though the hospital had an IV team of RNs who started or restarted IVs. The team leader was supposed to take a direct patient assignment also. Nursing students who were learning to give medications or new staff personnel being "oriented to meds" by the Inservice Department might take this function temporarily from a team leader.

The team leader went to the head nurse or charge nurse for advice or direction if necessary. For example, Vivian, an LPN team leader, had trouble deciding whether semicomatose Mrs. Georgetti should go for radiation therapy. Her respirations were rapid and she had a fever. Vivian went to the desk and asked Mildred, (the RN in charge that day) who did not go to the patient to make an assessment. Instead she said to Vivian, "Maybe she needs some oxygen. She went down the other day in worse condition." Mrs. Georgetti did go down for radiation therapy, and she died at five that afternoon.

When the researcher brought up this incident for discussion, the head nurse commented, "Once you establish a relationship with the doctors, they trust your judgment. I feel as if I have the trust of all of them. If I don't think a patient is well enough for radiation, I'll call them [Radiation], and when they [the doctors] come in, they'll say stop the radiation until further orders."

Team members were sometimes observed or heard comparing assignments, particularly if they felt they had more work than another team or if they thought the team leader was giving herself a lighter workload. Sometimes a team member was assigned one patient in a two-bed room, and a member from another team was assigned the remaining patient.

It was often observed by the staff that patients desired what their roommates got. Alice, the aide, said:

I have Mrs. Harris today in 225. But every time I go to do something for her, Mrs. Varney wants something. I don't like it when another staff person has a patient in the same room and then leaves her to me—this irritates me. I don't see why they don't care for their patients. ["They" referred to LPNs, RNs, and aide students.] They wash them and leave the patients for the day. I got so that I almost didn't want to go in the room to Mrs. Harris because I knew Mrs. Varney would ask me for something again.

"Can you talk about this to the staff?" asked the researcher.

"I'm not supposed to, but I do go right to the Rightway aide students, but they don't want to hear anything."

Students as Team Members

During the year, students from five programs with different learning objectives were assigned to EH II for a few hours, several days a week for two to four weeks of clinical experience. These programs included the Rightway aide program for adults with learning disabilities or emotional problems, the county vocational school's one-year practical nursing program, the county college's two-year associate degree program, the three-year Charles Hospital School of Nursing program, and the state university's four-year generic baccalaureate program. The head nurse was expected to select or recommend patients to be assigned to students in all of the programs except the associate degree program, whose faculty members assumed this responsibility. The focus of experience was different for each of the programs. For example, for the baccalaureate students the emphasis was to be on family stress, whereas the aide program emphasized training in basic bedside skills such as bathing and bed-making. The programs that prepared students for registered nurse licensure had an instructor on the unit; the other students had instructors who could be paged if they were needed.

The students were assigned to teams, but communication about their assignments was sometimes unclear. At times the staff viewed the aide students as a hindrance, because six extra bodies made the unit crowded.

Sometimes the lack of clarity about assignments resulted in two people doing one task or no one doing what was necessary. For example, Jill, the aide, said:

> Six Charles student nurses and their instructor were on the unit today, and several staff members complained that there was confusion of work allocation. Either the student nurses do not always know what they are supposed to do, or they just don't want to do it. Either way, the vital signs are often not obtained or patients don't receive their trays.

Alice, the other aide, mentioned that she continually checked up on the work of the students and filled in if they didn't do something that the staff expected them to do. A staff aide also noted that when more skilled students were taking care of patients, the staff became lax and missed call lights, thus breaking down patient-staff communication.

The Rightway aide instructor was observed on the unit assisting aide students with the direct physical care of patients or instructing them in post-mortem care. She went from unit to unit to supervise other groups of aide students. One afternoon at four-twenty, Karen, the head nurse, late getting off again, was stamping names on charts with the addressograph, and Jill was still there. Karen said, "This is one of the worst days." Sharon, an LPN, had called in sick, and Karen had switched Mildred to work on Thursday instead of that day because the unit was to have Rightway aide students. But, Karen said, "It was a poor judgment on my part." Jill said the Rightway students that day were more hindrance than help—"in fact, negligent."

"You mean like leaving side rails down?" the researcher asked.

"Worse than that," Jill said. "Like one spilled a bedpan in Mrs. Shumann's bed and was going to put a disposable Chux pad underneath her instead of changing the bed. I came in and saw the Rightway student looking guilty and asked her what happened."

The scope of experience for students was controlled to some degree by the nursing staff. For example, the Charles hospital school's instructor thought it unreasonable that Mildred "won't let senior students one month from graduation change an IV bottle, teach insulin injection to a patient, or allow practice in the team leader role." She commented, "It's a big jump from the responsibilities of the day before graduation to the day after."

Intrateam Conflicts

Team members also had difficulty with some team leaders. At conference one day, Alice and Jill, the aides, voiced their distress about working without a written assignment. Karen told them to discuss it with their team leader. "She is our team leader," they responded.

"I know who you mean," said Karen. "I'll talk to her." The aides were not optimistic about a change. They were referring to Libby MacGregor, the sixty-nine-year-old RN.

Jill said to the researcher:

It's difficult to work under Mrs. MacGregor. She doesn't like to make any assignments, and you don't know what you're responsible for. It's like "all in together girls." She says, "Let's start here and work our way around." But like I don't know what my duties are about getting vital signs in the morning and noon with her. The rule is that in the A.M. the team leader gets the blood pressure, and the aide gets the temperature. But at noon there is no rule—it's whoever seems to remember. But sometimes nobody remembers. Yesterday nobody got pressures on that whole side, and Mrs. Williams is really sick and on vital signs q. i. d. [four times a day] and they never got taken.

Jill thought the head nurse had an awareness of the problems but "sort of lets her [Mrs. MacGregor] go by. Consequently, by late morning," said Jill, "hardly any patients on our team are done." Jill added:

Libby kids about writing assignments. "Oh, phooey—that's the new way of thinking. I like to do my work and not waste all my time."

But it makes everybody's work harder for everybody on her team. I have to go around to see what hasn't been done. That's really bad. First it was care plans that she didn't want to write. Now she doesn't even want to write nurses' notes on the chart.

The researcher asked if Jill had talked to the head nurse. Jill felt she was in a precarious position as a new aide because the head nurse and Mrs. MacGregor "really get along very well. Karen thinks very highly of her." Jill's perception of the situation as somewhat unjust was demonstrated by her further comment, "I think even though she gives medications, I'm still overworked. When I see her out talking in the hall, it makes me feel like I've been treated unfairly."

Technicians and aides were not permitted to write on patients' charts or nursing care plans. The team leader was supposed to write down their assignments on an assignment sheet. By two in the afternoon the aides and technicians were supposed to have written down on the back of the assignment sheet any information they thought was pertinent about the patients. The team leader was then supposed to include pertinent comments in the nurses' notes.

A team member (aide) commented:

The nurses come to me at the patient's bedside for my report on the patients I've been assigned to or my written list and they want me to stand right there and give it. A person shouldn't hear that the man in the other bed was depressed today or any other part of the report. I have to steer them out in the hall. A lot has to do with the time schedule, but it only takes a minute to walk out. I notice that they don't pay enough attention to the patient's privacy in other ways. After the patients are here awhile they start not paying attention to draping the patients or pulling the curtains around the bed.

One thing that bothers me is how loudly the nurses speak. I guess it's after so many years of trying to overcome hard-of-hearing problems—they yell at everybody, especially the ones in pain—they flinch. Mrs. Kaiser has perfect hearing; she says she enjoys when I care for her because I don't yell at her and I'm patient. It's just I'm not raising my voice. Annette and Lisa don't, but Vivian, Mildred, and Libby do.

Role Blurring

There was much overlapping of activities of all role groups of the nursing staff. Aides did much of the direct patient care for even the sickest patients. Alice, for example, was assigned to Bill Kravitz and Flo Dunaway for the three days before their deaths. Both were forty-seven-years-old with extensive metastasis, including spinal involvement with considerable pain and loss of neurologic function.

Despite the fact that LPNs were not prepared by their programs to assume team leader role functions, they were used as team leaders interchangeably with RNs. Except for the RNs who were in charge in the head nurse's absence, the only distinctions between these two categories of workers seemed to be legal ones. According to the state's Nurse Practice Act, LPNs could not do certain role functions of RNs, such as administering intravenous heparin. For most of the year, the LPNs and aides formed the most stable group of employees, since after the departure of Annette and Lisa, most of the RNs worked part time.

This overlapping of role functions, particularly that of the team leader role, was not viewed as problematic by most staff. Annette commented on LPNs as team leaders:

Some RNs are very threatened. It doesn't bother me. There's always someone close by; they're not alone. They're not doing team nursing in the generic sense. But there's nothing in the LPN curriculum that prepares them for this role. That's a problem. I'm all for stimulating people and getting them to think patient awareness. As far as the planning of the care, they have no preparation for that.

Two of the LPNs felt that the team leader role was within their realm of responsibility. Vivian said, "LPNs are not given enough responsibility. We're qualified by our training," and Sharon commented, "It's the only thing that's manageable for an LPN. I could never run the floor."

The researcher questioned the head nurse about the lack of clear distinction between the utilization of RNs and of LPNs in direct patient care. Karen commented:

From the experience we've had with the RNs and LPNs, I guess I probably do put them in the same category. Some don't use the knowledge they have, and others are always seeking out further knowledge. I know there should be more of a distinction. My LPNs are exceptional. Some LPNs are more conscientious than some RNs. For example, Lisa doesn't take her responsibilities as seriously as the LPNs. She's more carefree and has a tendency to be forgetful at times.

Job commitment. It was the head nurse's view that the individual worker's motivation and specific commitment to the care of cancer patients were the major factors in the level of job performance, rather than the level of educational preparation. She cited the example of Clare Nelson, an evening-shift LPN in her midforties. "She became an LPN after she had radiation therapy to the spine [for a benign tumor] and a spinal fusion. She came here to work because she knows what it's like to be immobilized in a hospital bed for six months." The head nurse compared Clare with Ellen, a three-year hospital school graduate on the evening shift, by saying, "Ellen came here to work because it was the only job offer she got." She added:

> I compare Marlene Rush [LPN] with Vicki Martin [hospital school RN]. Vicki doesn't have the personal interest. She wanted a day job. June [part-time RN, A.S.] is the same. She doesn't have to work. She just does it to keep active. Marlene, in spite of several problems at home, any time of day you see her she is dedicated and busy. Alice [aide] came after her son died.

WORK ORDER

An elemental daily routine remained the only constant in a subculture that changed from day to day in activities, interpersonal relationships, and external influences from other departments. Patients were bathed and beds changed usually in the morning. Most diagnostic studies and therapies were done in the morning, and nurses carried out doctors' orders for medications and treatments. Meals were served three times a day. The afternoons, evenings, and nights were usually quieter since there was less movement of patients to and from the unit.

But all kinds of unpredictable events took place. For example, an informant told the researcher about Lynda Lacey, a twenty-three-year-old woman with kidney cancer and liver involvement, who was admitted with severe bleeding from the gastrointestinal tract and was recovering after transfusions. Her roommate, Mrs. Moss, was upset with Lynda because she kept the volume of her TV set too high, especially after nine at night, when the sets were supposed to be turned off. (Nurses did not enforce that policy as long as the volume didn't disturb other patients.) Mrs. Moss was also upset with Lynda's and her visitors' foul language and the fact that her boyfriend had been in bed with her the night before.

After these complaints, it was discovered that Lynda was missing from the unit, so staff and security were deployed to search for her. After an hour they found her on another ward visiting her sister. Some visitors expressed amusement that the staff did not know where their patients were. The staff, discussing the problem, "did not come up with a cure-all," but they decided "not to be judgmental." They also decided to safeguard the rights of the other patients and keep closer track of Lynda, said the informant.

Emergency admissions, deaths, doctors' rounds, different combinations of full-time and part-time nursing personnel each day, and changing conditions of patients made the unexpected the norm. For example, one morning, the three ladies in 217 had fecal impactions that had to be removed manually so their diarrhea could be controlled. Mr. Jacobs, who had been responding well to radiation treatment, died suddenly at four-thirty in the afternoon. Mrs. Brown had a severe transfusion reaction and was up all night with shaking chills, fever, and rash. Mr. Audoletto, who had lung cancer and brain metastasis, was walking in the hall with his family at eight in the evening but had a bronchial hemmorrhage and died at three the next morning. Mr. Dodwell, a confused elderly gentleman, needed to have a bowel movement but used a paper cup instead of the bedpan.

Mrs. McKenzie, who was very sick, died unexpectedly at four in the morning, and her eight children came in before six to view her body. A few weeks earlier their father had had a heart attack on EH II while visiting his wife, and he was still hospitalized on another unit. He had come to see his wife with some of their children the evening before she died, dressed in a business suit so she wouldn't worry about him.

Several patients, not realizing how weak they were and therefore not calling for assistance, fell getting out of bed or on their way to the bathroom, which necessitated calling a doctor to examine the patient and make out an incident report. A part-time night registered nurse, Paula Lynn, said to the researcher, "You should have come last week. Every room but one had an IV going—with one on the Holter pump. I'd like to know what's going on with some of these patients. I haven't had a chance to read the charts in two weeks."

The age of the patients and their degree of illness affected the work order also, since the staff was not enlarged when patients' needs for care increased. At one time, nineteen of the twenty-three patients required "complete care" in bed. At another time all the patients were over sixty and, in addition to cancer, had numerous other problems related to aging.

Legal Aspects

The work order could be interrupted by a call that required follow-up.

For example, one morning, a lawyer telephoned, and Annette spoke with him. He said he was representing Mr. Bailey, who was supposed to appear in court. He asked the nurse's name and asked if the patient could appear in court. Annette said, "No; the patient is confused." The lawyer asked if he could come into the patient's room and take a deposition; Annette again said, "No; the patient is confused and gets agitated easily." Annette heard clicks on the phone; it occurred to her that perhaps the conversation was being taped and that it was a lawyer for the other party in the case.

After Karen discussed this incident with the supervisor, a policy was set that any calls or visits from patients' attorneys must be screened by a member of the hospital administration. Nurses were not to give out any information over the phone to a patient's lawyer or to a doctor other than the patient's attending physician.

Karen said later that two patients on the unit were involved in lawsuits. One was involved in a workman's compensation case because he had sustained a pathologic fracture on the job. Another was suing her former physician regarding his misdiagnosis of her cancer.

Continuity Between Shifts

The three shifts appeared to function as separate though related subcultures. Each team leader from the day shift gave a report on her team's patients to the oncoming evening staff assembled in the conference room. Though the head nurse attempted to keep the same team with the same group of patients for one week, the work patterns of the part-time day nurses hindered the development of consistent groups or group leadership.

The fact that the head nurse never attended the afternoon report also lessened continuity. Since Karen made her rounds and rounds with doctors and was at the desk most of the day, she often possessed information that the team leader, occupied with a number of patients and staff, did not have. When the researcher asked Karen why she did not attend the report, she said: "During the course of eight hours the team leaders are at the desk several times, and I keep up. If there's a problem, I go in the room to check on it. They really don't report to me." Karen's absence also lessened a potential opportunity for staff development and accountability, since it was the researcher's observation that leaders reported in a fragmented, task-oriented way rather than using a nursing problem approach. Many of the staff LPNs and RNs who served as team leaders were in their first year of practice and were virtually unsupervised.

Rita, a new part-time staff nurse, commented during her orientation period, "Where I used to work, at the change-of-shift report we gave complete data on all patients, whereas here they only seem to report what happened on each shift.''

Karen replied, ''That's because most of the staff is full time and knows most of the patients.'' Actually most of the RN staff at this point were employed part-time.

The evening and night shifts followed a similar pattern of work allocation. There were two teams, each responsible for one end of the unit. On the evening shift, Pat, a full-time foreign-educated RN, was in charge. She was described as ''cold and distant.'' The researcher found her very uncommunicative. A holdover from the time when EH II was a self-care unit, Pat stated that she got no particular satisfaction from caring for cancer patients. She found it difficult to know what to say to ''emotional'' families and to care for patients with respiratory problems and unrelieved pain.

After visiting hours, a heavy emphasis was placed on medicating patients for sleep. Since Pat was in charge, the aides and Clare, the LPN, did much of the direct patient care, while Pat gave medications. Two of the aides were described as being ''afraid of dying patients.'' Clare's astute questions at reports, her active involvement in rehabilatation measures, such as getting patients to ambulate with her assistance, and her observations, made her stand out by comparison with other staff on the evening shift. For quite awhile the researcher mistakenly thought Clare was a registered nurse.

On nights, Catherine Vogel, an RN who worked two or three nights a week, stood out by comparison with the other staff on that shift. As Karen said:

> Catherine's exceptional; so is Clare Nelson. I'm not really impressed with Mrs. Lynn. She's been in a rut for too long. There's an emphasis on giving drugs to knock them out. That's the difference with Catherine. She sees that they get turned and talked to, too, and she'll be there to do it. Lynn misses a lot of important basic nursing things like a patient going a whole shift without voiding, a broken CVP manometer, and she closed off an ng [nasogastric] tube because the stuff was dripping out, instead of irrigating it or repositioning it.

The researcher asked Catherine one night how often she made rounds, since she was frequently away from the desk with a flashlight. ''Whenever I go down one wing to check a patient, I usually check them all,'' she said.

One night, Babe, a seventy-year-old aide, was out sick. Catherine said, ''She's terrific. I really miss her. She's the only one who can fix up Flo Hamill without hurting her.'' As Catherine was taking care of Flo later, Flo complained about the lack of care on the three-to-eleven shift. Catherine responded, ''Ask for Clare. She'll take good care of you.'' Many patients asked for Clare, and it was distressing to her when she was on the other team and couldn't possibly get to them because of the extent of her own assignment.

Shortly after the field work was completed, the researcher was told that because of a staff shortage on the evening shift, day RNs would be required to take their turn rotating to the evening shift. As a result of this new rule, June resigned and found part-time day work in a local general hospital. The staff agreed that Libby should be excused from the rotation. "I couldn't see a sixty-nine-year-old lady running this floor on three-to-eleven," Karen explained, adding, "Would you believe her husband didn't speak to her for a week when she told him she had to rotate?"

Time Themes

Though there was always a sense of time pressure, some individuals exhibited this more than others. Karen, the head nurse, was low-keyed, whereas when Mildred was in charge, she was perceived by staff to be the opposite.

Certain activities were expected to be accomplished within a certain period of time. A staff member's absence or long-term staff shortage caused concern that there were not enough workers to accomplish a set amount of work in a specified period of time. Care and charts had to be done so that the next shift could start its work on time and the staff could go off duty on time. Completing work on time was an expectation in role performance. Donna, an RN, B.S.N., who was having difficulty adjusting, said, "It takes me longer than anyone else to get done. But I don't see it as a problem. I see it as so what—eventually I get done. I have until three-thirty." But the staff saw it as a problem if a large part of her patients' care wasn't completed before lunch time.

Time was sometimes used as an excuse to avoid certain activities. For example, "Nursing care plans take too much time," or, "We don't have time for team conferences." Team conferences, an integral part of the team concept of planning for and evaluating nursing care of patients, as well as a method for learning about or reviewing the patients' medical conditions, were rarely held and were never observed by the researcher. Not only would these have offered a growth opportunity for the aides and technician, but it was evident that these persons who were most directly involved with the patients knew a lot about patients' problems, and there was no sharing of this vital information. It would certainly have increased the technician's and the aides' sense of worth.

Although lack of time was given as the reason for not holding team conferences, Annette said:

They're sporadic. Basically, care is given before lunch. You should be checking these patients in the P.M. anyway. It would be an appropriate time. But apparently a lot of people up here disagree with me. I do see that things are caught up. There seems to be a lull in the afternoon. Afternoons would be an ideal time. Last week we did one but that's sporadic. Tomorrow we're having students up here, and it would be a very good day to have a team conference.

"For the students' sake?" asked the researcher.

"No, for the people on my team to do a care plan. We're freer because we have the students," said Annette.

When p.r.n. (as needed) pain medication was not being given on time (that is, when the patient asked for it), Dr. Fisher responded in part by putting certain patients on a regular schedule for pain medication, such as every two or four hours. Standing orders were developed in part so that blood could be ready for patients to be transfused before the IV team left for the day.

Staff complained they did not have time to sit and talk with patients. The time when a patient wanted a staff person to listen frequently mismatched with a nurse's availability. "How can I sit and talk when I hear somebody throwing up in the next room?" a staff member asked.

After the researcher introduced herself to Catherine, the night nurse, and told her what the study was about, Catherine asked, "Do you talk to patients?" When the researcher answered affirmatively, she said:

Mrs. Dionne needs someone—she just started to open up. She asked me where I went to high school, and I told her Rochelle Academy. She asked if I commuted, and I told her I boarded. She asked me why, and I told her because my mother died when I was fifteen. She started to talk about her girls, they're fourteen and sixteen. Then the aide came to me for something for pain for Mr. Cirri, and I had to leave. I wish I had more time to talk to her.

The researcher went into Mrs. Dionne's room, but she had fallen asleep. One patient, who was in a talkative mood at a point in the day when a staff member had no time to sit, would give a clue that she could not talk later when time was available. An emesis basin beside her chin and a wan wave told anyone that Valerie Whelan had had her chemotherapy and wanted to be immobile, because any motion might start her vomiting and cause more pain in the area of her pathologically fractured rib.

Patients going to other departments for treatment interfered with the timing of activities on the unit. For example, t.i.d. (three times a day) medications were to be given at specific times: 10:00 A.M., 2:00 P.M., and 6:00 P.M. Lisa said one day, "Today every patient I went to give medicines to wasn't there." This problem seemed to lead the staff into violating one of the institution's and the state's norms: "The nurse is to remain with the patient until his medicine is taken unless otherwise written as a doctor's order." On the Oncology Unit, an antacid for patients on oral steroids, and viscous Xylocaine for relief of pain from radiation reaction in the tissues of the pharynx were often prescribed to be left at the bedside. But Annette said, after she had transferred to the Inservice Education Department:

> They are very lax on EH II; they have left medications with a confused patient. Sharon, the LPN, was never passed on meds but gives them anyway. She prepares medications too far in advance. One day I found a syringe of morphine in a patient's drawer. She signs meds as given before she gives them.

Ellen, a hospital-school graduate hired for the three-to-eleven shift, had to be passed on medications. One day she was being supervised on medications for the unit by an inservice instructor. At one-fifty in the afternoon she went into Mrs. Wiley's room with her two o'clock medications. Mrs. Wiley's daughter was visiting, and the patient was talking on the telephone. Ellen indicated to Mrs. Wiley that she had her medicines, but Mrs. Wiley ignored her and continued talking. Ellen waited. Mrs. Wiley's daughter suggested to her mother that she call the party back. Mrs. Wiley continued to talk until two-ten. Ellen had to give Mrs. Wiley an intramuscular injection (in the buttocks) but didn't realize that the patient was sitting on a bedpan, which had to be taken care of first. Ellen finally left the room at two-twenty and still had medicines to give the remaining seventeen patients. The instructor had been sitting in the hall waiting.

At one of Ted's conferences, at which staff were encouraged to express their feelings, Vicki, a first-year hospital school RN, said, "I hate these patients so much I want to go home. They're so slow taking their meds. I'm so mad at them that I feel like shoving the meds down their throats."

Mildred responded, "I'm glad you could say that, but take it under counsel, some could aspirate."

Ted tried to stimulate further discussion by asking Mildred, "Is it wrong to get angry?"

"That's a lousy question," said Mildred, closing off further discussion.

At another of Ted's conferences, the staff was talking about being rejected by some patients. June, a part-time RN, seemed to be rejected more often than the others. She said, "I get dirty looks from Mrs. Soules when I bring her medicine in."

"She gets mad at everybody," said Marlene.

"She's afraid she'll choke," said Mildred, adding, "She wants the nurse to stand there while she takes her medicine."

In a very low voice, Annette, who by this time was in the Inservice Education Department, said, "Everybody's supposed to wait [until the patient swallows his medicine]."

"But not everybody does," said Mildred.

NURSING CARE SYSTEMS

Despite the staff's good intentions, some common problems of hospitalized cancer patients were often not anticipated and not managed in any systematic way on EH II. Even the aides were aware of this. For example, the registered nurses recognized constipation as a common problem because of the effects of narcotics, immobility, change in diet, or neurologic impairment. They developed a bowel program, which they could initiate as a standing order. But there was a lack of communication, written and verbal, about which patients were to be put on the program and what their progress was. At conference, Alice said to the nurses, "If you [the team leaders] would tell us [the team members] when you give a patient on the bowel program a suppository, we could watch them more closely and put them on the commode or the bedpan so that results would be more effective."

With regard to pain, the researcher observed innumerable instances in which a patient's request for pain medication was relayed to the team leader, who prepared and took the medication to him or her without first assessing the patient's need for narcotic drugs as against other possible remedies for discomfort or complaint. One of the aides said:

> There is a lack of communications regarding p.r.n. meds for pain. If I go to the med nurse and say Mr. So and So needs medication, the med nurse doesn't write the request down, or there's so many people to get meds like around two o'clock that they might forget and the patient feels like they're not getting their adequate care. The delay depends on who's giving meds and how busy it is, like on weekends. I noticed certain patients who are more demanding will get it faster. It makes me encourage patients to ask for it. I asked for some for Mr. Michaelson, and he'd say they haven't come in yet. I'd go back fifteen minutes later, and he didn't get it. He was apologetic and too patient. I just tell him you ask everybody who comes in and even put your light on. Mr. Byren is fastidious; I don't know how he was raised, but he always has his pain on exactly three hours. He is on a regular schedule for pain medicine, but he always asks to make sure. Maybe at the point when I can give medicines, I'll be careful to write requests down. It's horrible to see them waiting for it.

Patient Education

Charles Hospital did not have a department of patient education or a patient education coordinator for the hospital. There were no printed explanations for patients about the tests they were to undergo, such as bone and liver scans, bronchoscopy, or gastroscopy. The only printed patient information observed on the Oncology Unit was a single instruction sheet on skin care to radiated sites, which was given to patients by the Radiation Therapy Department. The researcher first came across this on a patient's chart and asked the charge nurse why it was there. She said it should have been given to the patient, and would the researcher mind giving it to Mrs. MacTeague if she was going in there. Mrs. MacTeague had completed two and one-half weeks of a three-week course of radiation to the brain and said she had been washing her head with soap all along, contrary to the printed instructions.

Mr. Krivas had lung cancer, as well as a huge subcutaneous tumor in the subclavicular area that impinged on the nerves and caused a neuromuscular deficit in his right arm and hand. During the course of his radiation therapy, he developed thrombophlebitis in both legs. A small catheter was placed in a vein in his forearm for the intermittent administration (every six hours for several days) of heparin to lessen the chance of further clot formation. When Dr. Fisher told Mr. Krivas that the heparin catheter would be removed the next day, the patient said, "Is that what that's for? I thought I was getting chemotherapy."

Mildred was particularly interested in teaching families how to take care of the patient at home, such as procedures for bathing, toileting, preventing decubitus ulcers, and doing certain treatments. The doctors sometimes requested that family members be taught how to give an injection so they could give the patient pain medication at home, and the nurses would do this teaching. But there was no record in the nurses' notes that a teaching program had been started or that the family needed more instruction, and there wasn't any indication on the nursing care plan that a teaching program was in progress. The method for passing on this information to other shifts and to other teams was by word of mouth, which was frequently inconsistent and selective.

Mildred, who was actively looking for another job, thought the hospital needed a patient education coordinator, so she went to the director of nursing and proposed herself for the position. She was told there was no money for such a position in the budget. Mildred resigned from Charles two months after the conclusion of data collection.

Professional Standards

The Standards of Nursing Practice promulgated by the American Nurses' Association state systematically how nurses should assess client/patient status, plan nursing actions, implement the plan, and evaluate it, with reassessment and replanning if necessary. None of the nurses on the Oncology Unit or in the Inservice Education Department knew what the researcher was referring to when she asked them if, or how, they used the Standards of Nursing Practice.

At the start of the research year, the supervisor did start an audit system, "to see that the nurses' notes correspond with the nursing care plan as the Joint Commission wants." Weekly sessions were held with the EH II staff, working with one patient's chart. However, as the staff shortage persisted, these conferences were discontinued. After Annette transferred to the Inservice Education Department, the researcher asked the question again, "How are the Standards of Nursing Practice related to the 'real world' at Charles Hospital?"

Annette replied, "RNs are angry with the thinking aspect."

Nursing Care Plans

The outcome of planned patient care is supposed to be a set of directives or nursing orders, giving explicit direction to members of the nursing team caring for the patient. According to nursing department policy, plans were supposed to be initiated by the nurse who admitted the patient, further developed at team conferences with input from all team members, and updated by the team leader when indicated, again with input from others.

However, it was apparent to the researcher very early that the nursing care plans could not be relied upon. Some patients never had one done; some plans were attempted but incomplete; some were outdated. Generally, patient care was planned by the individual staff member assigned to a patient, and each staff member performed her assignment as she thought it should be done.

Nursing orders are supposed to carry the same significance for nursing care as doctors' orders do for medical care. According to the principles of team nursing, the identified nursing problems and orders (approaches) are to be written on a nursing care plan on the patient's Kardex. The Charles Nursing Policy Manual states:

> A nursing care planning conference is held daily for each team. The conference and the patient to be discussed should be planned in advance and noted in the assignment sheet. The result of the conference should be placed on the Nursing Care Plan on the Kardex.

Written plans for nursing care were done only if there was time after everything else was done. Occasionally, the head nurse would write "Nursing Care Plans" on the assignment sheet, indicating it was a specific assignment for teams that day. The fact that they were a chore and a burden to some was illustrated by Marlene Rush, who commented one day as she sat down at the desk, "Nursing care plans, I hate them, I hate them."

Much of the impetus for written care plans being a required part of patient care came from outside agencies. For example, during the first month of data collection, the head nurse attended a Charles' head nurses' meeting and then reported to her staff. She told them that the JCAH report, following their recent survey of Charles Hospital, stated that the nursing notes and nursing care plans were "60 percent improved" over what they had been on the last accreditation visit, but that 60 percent improvement was still not an acceptable level and that a revisit would be made.

Later, on an unannounced visit to Charles, a state department of health inspection team found nursing care planning to be deficient. At a staff meeting, Karen said, "Nursing care plans seem to be a chore. Everyone should take part. You should be doing care plans from the admission data base."

Since there did not seem to be much improvement in care plans after these meetings, the researcher asked the staff about them. Julie, the technician, said, "I'm not using very much. I don't have much time to do that. We're given an assignment like this [written]. I try to see the Kardex, not so much the nursing care plan."

Jill, an aide, commented, "I've sat in the conference room a few times when they're writing on the care plans. It does take quite a bit of time."

"Do you use them?" asked the researcher.

"I need them," said Jill, adding, "There's one on Mr. Sample. He's been here awhile. But there's none for Mr. Landes and Mr. Kravitz. Annette is by far the best care plan writer. Mrs. MacGregor has no leave for care plans, and she'll tell you all about it."

When the researcher asked Libby MacGregor about the use of nursing care plans, she responded:

> Don't get me involved with that. That's the one thing I refuse to do. I guess I'm too practical. I like facts to deal with. I don't like compositions. My nurses' notes are short and sweet. You haven't got time to read all the stuff on the Kardex.
>
> Sometimes you have time to sit down and read the notes, but sometimes you don't have time.
>
> If I had a choice, I'd like to have an assignment and take care of my patients but not be team leader.

Yet Mrs. MacGregor worked only three days a week and frequently complained that it was hard to get information about the patients she was assigned to after being away several days. She did not seem to recognize that a written care plan could provide information that would be helpful to her and the patient.

It was evident at a staff conference that only Annette and Lisa had the basic preparation necessary for this responsibility. The researcher attempted to help at one audit conference by suggesting that a generality about a patient's fluid intake be restated as an order—how much fluid, what type, how frequently, what specific times, with what assistance. This suggestion was not perceived as helpful, because they were writing the plan for three days retrospectively, and the patient's needs had changed; his condition had improved. The researcher suggested perhaps there was no longer a problem. But Karen, the head nurse, said, "Look, our problem is to write something down." To the supervisor she said, "You had the course on nursing care planning; I didn't."

At a conference with Charles' senior nursing students, their instructor said:

Students can't rely on nursing care plans and therefore don't use them. Students write nursing care plans, and then the staff doesn't use them. We would like to see students get a report from the nursing care plan. Even Kardexes are not always updated. A patient whose diet was marked clear liquid was supposed to be fed an egg. The nursing care goal for Mrs. MacTeague was written "to reduce abdominal distention," but that's a medical problem which she's had for three years. The other night they removed 3,300 cc of ascitic fluid.

One of the students thought the nursing care plans on EH II were much better than on the other floors, adding, "A lot of the other floors don't have them at all."

Another student said, "Those admission nursing history forms here at Charles are too much. You ask them [patients], 'What are your daily habits?' 'Shower at night.' 'Well, I'll write that down, but here you're going to get a bath in the morning.' " When the researcher suggested that the staff on EH II would try to arrange for the patient to shower at night, the student responded, "Other floors wouldn't put up with a patient washing at night."

A senior student said, "I'd like to write down the little ditty things that patients tell me are important to them."

The instructor said, "Well, what's a nursing care plan?"

"Write down the little ditties?" the student asked.

Prior to the start of data collection, the supervisor, Frances, had started to write a series of standard care plans specific to oncology patients, but she "had to let it drop for lack of time." During a discussion of a JCAH site visit, the head nurse told the researcher that nurses don't have time to get to the patients' nursing care plans.

Mildred added:

Yes, like mine of Mr. Taylor. I've been off for four days. On Friday when I admitted him, he was comatose and he looked so bad that I wrote, "See standard care plan for terminally ill patients" on his care plan. But today he's the most active patient in his room.

When the researcher had gone into the room early in the day on rounds with Mildred, she had been shocked to see Mr. Taylor sitting on the side of his bed bathing himself. His only complaint was about his hemorrhoids. The researcher asked the head nurse later what she thought was responsible for the man's marked improvement. She shrugged and said,

"Possibly rehydration."

On one occasion the staff was elated. When Lisa and Annette had taken a "difficult" patient, Mr. Christoforo, into the conference room and written a care plan with him, he had added a problem that neither of the nurses had identified—gas. Previously, Alice, the aide, had said, "Christoforo—I can't get anywhere with him. He's all in himself." But several days after Lisa and Annette did the care plans with him, Alice said, "They did him good to talk with him about his care plan. Today, he's talking easily about his colostomy."

Later in the year, after observing several times that the head nurse didn't take the charts or Kardex (including nursing care plans) on rounds with her, the researcher asked her how she did use nursing care plans. Karen said:

> I don't use them too much, to be truthful. I guess it's that I'm not oriented to them enough yet to use them as a helpful tool in nursing, and I guess it's because the plans don't get done until the patient's been there for awhile—you know the problems when they come in—I know they would be a good tool for report or making up the assignments each day. But we just haven't gotten that far yet. It will take a while. The busier we are, the less they get done. They are so hung up on taking care of patients' physical needs that they feel as though a nursing care plan isn't necessary for them. They are lowest in priority, especially shift to shift.

> You have one nurse [Libby MacGregor] who refuses to do them. She certainly gets told about it often enough. Yesterday I said, "Everyone who can write care plans [meaning all RNs and LPNs] has to write one today." Libby said, "I can't write care plans." But to top it off, the supervisor came up and wrote her care plan for her.

Karen added that Mrs. MacGregor "gives excellent nursing care. I don't think she is the best team leader in the world, but she has common sense that a lot of young people lack." Karen thought this common-sense knowledge "makes up for some of the other things Mrs. MacGregor lacks." But, Karen added:

> With nursing care plans—Libby's closed her mind to them entirely. They're worthless and useless to her. If she sees somebody writing and patients are not being fed, dentures not being removed for mouth care, she gets angry. "There's too much paper work in nursing," she says.

After Annette transferred to the Inservice Education Department, the researcher asked for her views about written nursing care plans on EH II. Annette said, "I don't honestly know of one person on that floor who uses care plans. When they do write them, they do it because the state wants them to."

"Is there a reason?" the researcher asked.

"No one has come up with an answer why they're not used. We need more inservice about nursing care plans," Annette added.

Thus several factors contributed to the lack of progress in writing more specific care plans for patients. These included the RNs' and LPNs' lack of preparation in the nursing process; undeveloped writing skills; lack of acceptance of their value on the unit, because of the lack of a problem-solving approach to nursing practice in their basic nursing socialization process, reinforced by the Inservice Education Department, which did not provide consistent instruction; lack of time; lack of accountability, except that imposed by outside accrediting agencies; and lack of space and milieu for quiet reflective thinking.

State Inspection

In January an inspection team from the state department of health arrived at the hospital unannounced. (Some of the nurses thought that Dr. Jones had summoned them, but there were unannounced visits to other hospitals in the area also.) Mildred was in charge of the unit at the time, and an informant said that when the news reached her via the hospital grapevine, she gave four directions to the staff:

Lock the unused drawers on the medicine carts.
Lock the medicine room door.
Keep all linens off the floor.
Clear all IV bags off the counter at the nurses' station.

The informant continued:

Since all these four procedures were the exact opposite of what we usually do, the staff had to continually correct themselves as they automatically did the wrong thing. The staff made many comments about how inconvenient this was, but they were relaxed enough to be able to joke about it.

The inspectors did not come to EH II that day, but, the next day the staff was tense because they expected the inspectors. Some of the other units had "gotten into trouble" because they were letting LPNs give fractional doses of narcotics and because their nursing care plans were "scanty." The head nurse reminded the staff to observe the four temporary norms.

The LPNs on EH II had been figuring out and giving fractional doses of narcotics, especially morphine. The head nurse thought it was unreasonable that they were not supposed to do so, because they could figure out the doses as well as RNs. One of the LPNs said, "It seems strange that the hospital insists the LPNs take a pharmacology course which stressed the calculation of fractional dosages, and then the state doesn't permit them to calculate."

That day a student LPN on the unit told one of the aides that she noted that the nurses on EH II did not stay with patients until they had taken their medication, but left them at the bedside, not checking to see that patients had taken them. She said the unit would be reprimanded if the state found this out, but both were "afraid" to tell this to anyone in authority on the unit.

When the inspection team arrived on EH II, they selected at random a patient's chart and the corresponding nursing care plan. It happened that the patient, Mrs. Golden, had been transferred to EH II from North 5 two days before. Frances said, "All kinds of things had happened, errors included, but they did not occur on EH II." Frances and Karen spent an hour and a half with the inspectors, trying to track down the source of the errors and make plans for dealing with them. The patient had come to EH II without a nursing care plan, and the staff hadn't gotten around to doing it yet.

Since EH II was primarily a medical oncology unit, the staff did not have much experience with patients who had been treated surgically for head and neck cancer. Mrs. Golden, who was transferred to Dr. Long's care, had been admitted for reconstructive surgery of the jaw, but her bone scan had revealed questionable metastasis below the prospective surgical site on the lower jaw. This turned out to be a "deep-seated infection," which cleared with an antibiotic research protocol. Mrs. Golden had cancer of the floor of the mouth and had had a radical neck dissection four months earlier and a gastrostomy. It was difficult to understand her speech, and she secreted a great deal of saliva, which drained constantly from her mouth. She also had a dressing on her neck. The informant told the researcher that the team leader was unable to find any information on the chart about the type of dressing to be placed on Mrs. Golden's neck or the kind of mouth care she should receive. The nurses' notes were terse and unhelpful, and the doctor's orders did not specify anything. Much time was spent waiting for a doctor to look at the neck incision and then trying to decide what had been done in the past and what to do from then on. When staff did find out, they communicated her care by word of mouth rather than through a written nursing care plan.

Mrs. Golden remained on EH II for many weeks and during that time had two surgical procedures. One day, in Dr. Fisher's presence, her surgeon commented that Mrs. Golden got such good care on EH II, he would like to admit more of his patients there. This threat to territoriality caused Dr. Fisher's facial expression to change, but he said nothing. After the surgeon left, Dr. Fisher indicated that he wasn't in favor of EH II becoming a surgical cancer unit and said to Karen, "Can he do that?"

"Do what?" Karen asked.

"Admit more surgical patients here? What are the rules? What's written down?"

"I don't know," said Karen.

Role Conflict

Nurses with BSNs who had specific preparation for the leadership role (Annette and Donna) did not necessarily meet professional role expectations. Donna had considerable difficulty adjusting to the unit and asked to be relieved of team leader responsibilities. Annette, who was highly respected as a team leader, sometimes yielded her professional values for those of the work situation.

For example, Mrs. Margolis, an elderly woman from the opposite side of the state, lived in a trailer court with her retired husband. She had become Dr. Long's patient when her daughter had lived in the area, but she had since moved away. "It costs me thirty-seven dollars a visit to Dr. Long and ten dollars for someone to drive me," she said. After she was admitted to the hospital, her husband couldn't visit more than once a week because of the cost of transportation. Someone had given Mrs. Magolis the business card of a doctor in her own area, but when she asked Dr. Long what he thought of that doctor, "he threw the card at me. 'He's no cancer doctor,' he said," spouted Mrs. Magolis. She had reason to be angry, but she often took her angry feelings out on the nursing staff. Julie, the timid technician, incurred her wrath by suggesting that Mrs. Margolis could do some of her own care. Mrs. Margolis said of Donna, "I don't like Donna. She walks like she has a load in her pants." Mrs. Margolis, who was receiving radiation therapy for spinal metastasis from breast cancer, had a number of physical and psychological problems, but nothing was written on her care plan. As team leader, Annette assigned herself to Mrs. Margolis and two other bedfast patients in the same room. She was also responsible for supervising the patients to whom Alice, the aide, was assigned, and for medications, injections, and treatments for all of the team's patients. For a number of days, Alice had taken care of Mrs. Margolis and the other two patients as her only patient assignment, and since Mrs. Margolis had no visitors, Alice had done her personal laundry. When Annette took over, Mrs. Margolis started asking her early in the day to do her wash. Annette explained that she would get to it, but that she had to do medications first. The woman kept sending messages to the desk, putting her light on, and expressing her annoyance verbally to Annette. "That really bugs me," said Annette. "I told her I'd do it. The trouble is she had Alice for a few days, and Alice had time to do all the niceties. I told her I'll get to the wash and I will." Annette did the wash late in the afternoon.

At one of Ted's conferences, Annette again stated how much that "bugged" her. Alice, the aide, said, "Annette, any time you run into a situation like that I'll be glad to do the wash."

The researcher asked the head nurse about the situation. "It's Annette's own fault. She made out the assignment. She shouldn't have assigned herself to those patients."

Later the researcher asked Annette, "Did you think of assigning the aide to do the wash, and you do Mrs. Margolis' nursing care plan since she has none and is having a number of problems?"

"No. It's important for the aides to know that nothing is beneath you. They've had their problems on this floor with nurses who don't carry their fair share."

"You did so well with Mr. Christoforo's plan," the researcher commented.

"Well, she [Mrs. Margolis] can't come to the conference room."

"Can't you take the Kardex to her bedside?" asked the researcher.

"Oh, I never thought of that," said Annette.

STAFF DEVELOPMENT

None of the staff had long-term, formalized preparation in oncology nursing. The supervisor and head nurse had attended a week-long oncology nursing course and had observed at cancer hospitals, and a few of the staff RNs and LPNs had attended one-day nursing sessions sponsored by the local unit of the American Cancer Society. Lisa, an RN, and Vivian, an LPN, reported to the staff about such a workshop, but their reports were casual impressions without significant content or orderly presentation. Occasionally, the head nurse or supervisor or one of the staff nurses would recommend an article she had read in a nursing journal to other staff members. There was no specific course of instruction for new staff about the disease of cancer, its treatment, or nursing care. A new member of the nursing staff would be given several Xeroxed articles on cancer treatment to read and perhaps some cassette tapes on death and dying from the medical library. There was no plan to assess the self-study or the on-the-job learning of a new staff member, though several had been out of active nursing for many years.

Staff education in the nursing care of cancer patients was not identified as a role function by the supervisor, head nurse, or Inservice Education Department staff. The head nurse stated her concern about this on several occasions. Once the researcher asked her if the plans for the Oncologic Unit in the new building included an office for her so that she could withdraw to do some thinking and planning without all the distractions of the present nurses' station. She said, "I didn't have a thing to do with the plans. I hope they hire a clinician for Inservice Education."

Inservice Education taught new staff on the unit the technique of administering medications but did not teach the theory relevant to the nursing responsibilities of drug administration. In fact, this department overlooked some readily accessible learning opportunities. For example, on a bulletin board directly opposite the department's office were posted brochures announcing the week's N.C.M.E. (Network for Continuing Medical Education) video-cassette program, including a self-assessment quiz, which could be viewed in the library. Though Inservice staff had to pass this announcement daily, they did not further publicize such offerings as "Terminal Cancer: The Hospice Approach to Pain Control" or "Terminal Cancer: The Hospice Approach to the Family." After the researcher viewed these programs in the library and noted that the staff on EH II could utilize, some of the principles of care, she called them to the head nurse's attention. Some of the staff were able to view the programs, but due to the time pressures of the work situation, there was no group discussion or sharing of information afterward.

Dr. Long said that he had been interested in educating nurses on such subjects as chemotherapy. "But," he said, "I gave up. I'd start lecturing with nine in the room and end up with one. They all got up and left." The staff nurses said that when they attended class in the conference room, there were not enough people taking care of the patients, and they had to leave to get certain things done on schedule. Moreover, they could not concentrate well when they were concerned with meeting patient care needs on time.

Many of the staff voiced their concern about lack of inservice education. Lisa said:

> If I were in charge of this floor, I would have conferences all the time on all phases of oncology. There's not enough teaching for us or the patients. Patients ask questions about rads and how their dose is figured out. I don't think many of the staff can answer them. I think patients should be aware of what they have to deal with with their own bodies rather than say, "Here's my body, do something with it, fix it."

Mildred commented:

> This place is very routine. There's just not enough writing or education going on. That bothers me. They're all getting these management degrees. The thing I'm interested in is physician's assistant, where you field for the doctor. I've asked Dr. Fisher to teach us to listen to heart and lung sounds.

Clare, on the evening shift, said, "There is not enough help, and there's too much paperwork. The lack of continuing education upsets me. I asked the inservice instructor if I could use the library to get some things on my own."

Jill, the aide, had worked on the unit for two weeks when she attended one of Ted's conferences, which took place after Annette announced that she was leaving the unit for the Inservice Education Department. Lisa was leaving the unit also. Ted asked, "What do you think we can do to get Annette to stay?"

Jill recalled that some of the staff thought that an improved work situation might entice Annette to stay.

Somebody said, "Let's not talk about death. Let's talk about the floor not being specialized enough." We were all supposed to write down five suggestions to improve the floor and bring them to conference in two weeks. I took that seriously, and I wrote mine down. Everybody else laughed and said they're not important. That upset me a little. If they have complaints, they should write suggestions.

Four of Jill's suggestions, after two weeks of employment, were:

1. Improve communication with patients. Staff should be more open to using the word "cancer." Nurses tend to avoid using it.

2. There should be more opportunity for inservice education for nursing staff to update themselves and keep alert.

3. Contact cancer units in other hospitals to get ideas about handling problems such as diet for patients who have GI upset [diarrhea, vomiting] from chemotherapy or radiation therapy.

4. Do nursing care plans. Some patients have been here a long time, and nothing has been written. Aides need nursing care plans.

Mildred refused to make a list, saying, "I'm upset with the way these conferences are going. I'm not getting anything out of them. That material (improvement of the work situation) is for the head nurse and supervisor to handle."

Lisa didn't do one because she was annoyed that Ted focused on Annette's resignation. "Anyone who knows her knows that this move is part of her long-range career goals. It had nothing to do with the staff or the work on the unit."

Dr. Fisher, who was president of the local unit of the American Cancer Society, was credited with arranging for full scholarships from the society for two nurses to attend a national conference on cancer nursing held in the Midwest in the late spring. Karen received one of the scholarships, along with Marge, the nurse in the Radiation Therapy Department. Midge, Dr. Fisher's office nurse, also attended. The researcher attended in order to get a broader perspective on the field of oncology nursing; she was pleased to meet the others at the conference and enjoyed their company.

All three nurses found the three-hour opening session "boring," in which several nationally recognized nurses discussed concepts, issues, and trends in cancer nursing and cancer nursing education. Other conference sessions focused on the subjects of pain, bioethics, and rehabilitation. It was possible to attend only two of these three conferences, and the three Charles nurses chose to attend the same two conferences in a group; none of them attended the very significant session on bioethics. None attended an impromptu session on nursing research on cancer units. Later, Karen asked if she could borrow the researcher's tapes so that she could make a set of tapes for the EH II staff.

After Annette transferred to Inservice Education, there were more staff education offerings on EH II, dealing mainly with techniques, such as sites for intramuscular injection, and demonstrations of equipment. A slight change of emphasis from skills to concepts was made with the scheduling of a class for aides on "The Hostile Patient."

Annette experienced some conflict concerning her new role as inservice instructor for EH II and her former role as staff nurse there. When two male patients in one room were disoriented for a week (both recovered and became mentally clear), the stress of this type of assignment came up for discussion at Ted's conference, at which Annette was present.

Karen said, "I'd rather they wouldn't talk. I'd go crazy."

Mildred asked, "How do you cope? I joke."

Karen responded, "That wouldn't be my choice."

Mildred added, "I have this affliction that I have a motor mouth. If they say it's too bad it's rainy, I'll agree with them, even if it's a beautiful sunny day. I just talk to them in the same context they talk to me."

Though the researcher understood that the sessions with Ted were to help staff deal with their feelings rather than for instruction, she asked Annette later if she planned to initiate any education sessions on the care of temporarily disoriented patients, since there is a body of knowledge on reality orientation and therapeutic ways of dealing with confused patients. Annette responded:

> I'm on the outside looking in. I didn't realize before how they did cope—I was concerned with myself. If there is a need—and I'm not sure there is—I wouldn't be the one to do it. I could suggest it. I would need it just as much as they would. I don't think I could feel comfortable that just because I had the time to read a book or research, I could present it and say this is how it should be done—I was part of that.

WORK STRESSES

Nursing staff who worked in this subculture were subject to infection from sputum, wound, and abscess drainage and from vomitus and feces. The supervisor noted that almost every staff nurse got an upper respiratory infection shortly after starting work on the unit. The staff stood or walked on a hard-surfaced floor for most of the eight-hour shift, and there was constant risk of back injury from lifting, turning, or supporting heavy patients. There was also the risk of physical injury from disoriented, combative patients and the physical fatigue from almost constant activity.

The researcher planned her evening and night experiences on the unit for January and February. The severity of the winter weather conditions gave her renewed appreciation of the hazards the nursing staff faced in getting to or from work at eleven at night in a snowstorm or having to be on the road before six in the morning in near-zero weather.

The number of patients with dying trajectories affected the staff also. Not only was the physical care difficult, but on three occasions during the year, there were four deaths within three or four days, which added considerable emotional strain. Patients' personalities and their coping difficulties affected the staff, too. As Sharon said, "Some days you can have two patients and be more exhausted from the emotional part of it than the physical exhaustion that comes from caring for six to eight other patients."

Vivian said, "If we have a lot of sick patients with unrelieved pain, it seems to me like it affects the staff, and that it is a down day. I'm a coward as far as pain is concerned. I just don't know how to deal with it." Annette commented:

Take Mrs. Harris. She's been back many times. A very beautiful woman, always well groomed. To see her like this, it's draining.

The people you have seen come in again and again. . . . They come in like anyone else on the street, and then there's the last time. . . .

It continues to shock you. You never get used to it. And every patient's course is different with what they have and how they cope.

While the staff understood that a stage of anger is part of the patient's coming to terms with his own mortality, they had considerable difficulty coping with anger directed at them and with rejection by angry patients. For example, Mr. Charleston, a forty-nine-year-old man with lung cancer, was described as "irritable, depressed, doesn't want to be bothered, and angry." His mother took his cigarettes away, because he was smoking while the respiratory therapist was giving him his IPPB (Intermittent Positive Pressure Breathing) treatments. He made comments to June like, "Don't ask stupid questions," and "Get the hell out of here." He upset Sharon when he refused to be bathed or shaved for several days. He told her there was "too much poking around and no hope for specific problems." She said at evening report, "All he wants is a gun to be left alone and shoot himself. He says, "It's terrible to go through this alone.'"

A few days later Mr. Charleston asked Sharon to give him a bath and shave him. She reported, "There's a big change in his disposition." She admonished the group at the three o'clock report, "Don't do anything to him, or you'll answer to me. If he drinks 1,000 cc per shift, Dr. Long will send him home. Today he took in 705 [cc]."

When June mentioned that she was rejected by Mr. Vincent, everybody moaned. "There's not much you can do for him. He got his wife so upset the day he came in that we had to take her to the exit in a wheelchair," said Karen.

One day Rita came to Ted's conference very discouraged. Recently remarried and new to the area, she had been working on the unit a short while. Her seventeen-year-old daughter had just decided to leave her mother and return to live with her remarried father. Rita was grieving over this loss and also having difficulty adjusting to the Oncology Unit. She described how Mr. Kravitz had overtly rejected her, inferring that he was better off without her. Nothing seemed to satisfy him, and she felt frustrated and useless.

Mr. Kravitz was a forty-seven-year-old diabetic with multiple myeloma and increasing neurologic deficit from spinal cord involvement. When he was first admitted, his brother came at visiting hours and walked him up and down the hall after he had had a rod inserted in his humerus for treatment of a pathologic fracture. Mr. Kravitz' disease was progressive. While on the unit, he lost control of his bladder and bowel function and had seizures, severe nausea, vomiting, and pain. Rita said:

> I know patients go through stages of grief, including anger; and I make myself available to them. But Mr. Kravitz . . . he's so mean. I find it hard to be firm, but some things, like injections, are necessary. I'm trying to help them, and they don't want my help.

Some of the staff gave suggestions. "Respect them," said Karen.

"Come back in a couple of hours, and they may be ready," suggested Vivian.

When Mr. Kravitz was first admitted, he had heard Mr. Long, his roommate, say to Dr. Fisher, "Just slowly take away the IV and let me die."

Mr. Kravitz said to Jill, "I can't understand that. As long as I have any hope, I'll keep going." He also told Jill, "The nurses are coming in more often now because I have a decubitus." He said he was sitting in a wet bed for long periods of time, and no one checked him. He didn't ask to have the bed changed.

Mr. Kravitz died two weeks before his roommate, Mr. Long. At Ted's next conference, after Mr. Kravitz died, the researcher asked Rita for some follow-up about her relationship with him. She said, "Oh, we got on well, on much better terms. He even apologized for being impatient with me."

Vivian interrupted and said that she had been talking with the pathology lab worker who assisted at Mr. Kravitz's autopsy. Vivian added, "The assistant said he didn't know how Mr. Kravitz wasn't screaming all of the time—he had tumors on top of tumors and pathologic fractures of both arms and back." The researcher watched Rita's facial expression—this was difficult for her to hear.

Ted asked the group if they ever felt guilty when they were the target of a patient's anger. Karen described a situation in which a daughter, who had been with her mother all night, got angry because she wasn't called to be there when the mother died. "She would have just gotten home, and it was hard to predict when the mother would die because she had been dying for days. I felt guilty at first, but then it went away. It goes away faster now than it did when I first came to the unit."

Mildred said, "Mine disappears when I get home. I have to get to a different environment."

"How about you, Annette?" asked Ted.

"Well, I don't feel guilty. I'm human, and we all make mistakes," Annette commented.

Cumulative stress at certain times resulted in a shared sense of frustration. Alice said at one of Ted's conferences, "You never sit down, and you never feel that you've done enough. We go home late every night, and I'm too tired to do anything else. At least tonight I don't have to go home smelling like doo-doo."

Vicki complained, "The patients want you to sit down and talk with them, and you don't have time," and Marlene added, "The biggest frustration is lack of staff to give the care I would like to give."

Ted often tried to reassure the staff that they were providing a worthwhile service. One day he asked the group, "What do you give and what do you get?"

Annette offered:

> Some days you give and you give and you give, and nothing is good enough. Like with Mrs. Wiley and Mrs. Margolis. Both needed lots of strokes. But nurses need strokes, too. There are certain times when every patient you have gives you no strokes at all. I need encouragement—not much—like when you've cared for a patient, and you see the light doesn't go on as often as previously, that's fine. I'll take any sign, verbal or nonverbal.
>
> But when I have done my damnedest, and things get said. . . . With Mrs. Wiley, you could do cartwheels backward—it was either wrong or wasn't enough. I say to her, "What is it I can do for you?" I'm lost as to what road to take. Then she'd go into her medical history again. I know it's reasonable to have such patients respond in this way, but your ability to cope on certain days is limited. Even a roommate who gives strokes would balance it out, but some days you get nothing.

Dr. Fisher told the researcher he spent three times as much time at Mrs. Wiley's bedside as at any other patient's. Mrs. Wiley's brother was a physician in the Midwest, and she frequently telephoned him for advice. Annette suggested that sometimes patients' families "want to hang the blame on the nurse. Like when Mr. Tindall died, there were about twelve relatives around, and not one of them said anything to me; but they all looked like they were blaming me. I sound paranoid, don't I. Well, I felt paranoid [giggle]."

Another day, the researcher passed the head nurse in the hall. She seemed exasperated. The researcher then went in to see the usually quiet Mrs. Dodwell, who was angry and said she had been "suffering since early this morning. The doctor ordered something for pain, and I haven't gotten it yet." The researcher checked the schedule and told Donna, the team leader, about the complaint. Donna said that Dr. Long never ordered anything until just then, which was about two-thirty. By three o'clock Mrs. Dodwell was crying because she had had burning on urination after her Foley catheter was taken out in the morning. In addition, she said she was freezing. "I'm going home—I'm calling an ambulance. It's freezing in that room."

Donna, stating this at report, added, "Mrs. Voltz in the same room said she couldn't stand it and wants to get out of here." She added, "Nursing care stunk today. We were just understaffed. It's me and Jill on that side—that's all. I'm doing IVs, medications, enemas, and colostomy irrigations." (Jim Jason was being prepped for surgery.)

The staff also became angry at family members. Alice said of Mrs. Wenke, the wife of a patient:

> She writes notes in a book about all the things we're not doing. She won't give her husband a glass of water because she says the nurses are paid. She was angry yesterday because he didn't have a bath, but he was down in X-Ray for five hours. She compares the performance of staff members. Sometimes they have more time to do the little things and then she expects that all the time. She gets him upset. She says, "I'm going to spout my mouth off." He mimics her. "She's going to spout her mouth off." She even has Clare Nelson upset on evenings.

> We all do our best.

Mr. Ralph, eighty years old, had cancer of the floor of the mouth, which was treated with radiation. He was readmitted dyspneic and irritable with pneumonia. He recovered and eventually was discharged, but the staff found him difficult. Sharon said:

> He's grumpy. He's not supposed to smoke; he not only smokes, but he sits in front of the oxygen tank at his bedside and deliberately blows the smoke in the direction of the outlet valve. We finally got him to smoke in the hall, but he won't use an ashtray. He just drops the ashes wherever they fall.

Some patients were angry at staff over specific events. When the researcher went to see Rachel Brown, Mrs. Allen had just been admitted to the same room. Mrs. Brown said her roommate was really upset because she had heard Mildred refer to her as a "pain in the ass" when she asked the nurse to recheck her diet order. Mrs. Allen had been told to drink lots of fluid because she was getting chemotherapy and didn't understand that she could eat, too. She wouldn't take Mildred's word and wanted her to check the doctor's order. Mrs. Allen said, "I'm really angry with her. She needs something—to be married or something."

The researcher suggested to Annette that patients could be angry at staff members for real or perceived inadequacies in their care. "How does staff assess the basis for the patient's anger rather than simply ascribing it to a stage in the dying process?"

"Everybody does their own assessment in their own head," Annette replied.

There were no planned classes or consultation services to help staff understand patients' behavior, their own responses, or appropriate nursing intervention. Some staff members recognized that others were not coping adequately. For example, one aide stated:

> If I could be idealistic, I would hand-pick the people to work on this floor, and the others I would get rid of. Vivian, she has a very negative attitude, which is half the battle; she's very impatient with the patients. She'll almost yell at them when it's not necessary. She's lax in giving treatments in that she'll delay aspirating somebody. I'll say, "We should Posey this man," and she'll say, "Don't worry about it." She makes me feel like I don't know anything. She even makes some of the RNs feel inadequate, like Donna. Maybe she should be on a floor where you don't need as much patience. And it's not a racial thing either. And I know I'm right. Some of the patients say to me, "Boy, I don't like it when that lady comes." And I don't think it's a color problem either. She just comes across very gruffly.

> Julie [the technician] has a sour attitude. She's insecure, you can tell when she is—she emits a high-pitched laugh; when she's criticized, it's a caustic laugh.

The researcher asked Annette, "What do you do about a patient's anger?"
She answered:

> I try to get objective data. I ask them when they first started feeling angry. I try to check out what they say with the Kardex, notes, asking the people involved, and if I can't find out, then I will tell the patient. Some people I will confront. If they start expressing anger about generalizations, and I've tried to check out what they've said and I can't, I'll say, "You're not angry at us, you're angry at something else." Mrs. Storey was a good one. She had a lot of anger. She was so furious one night that she scared the three-to-eleven and night staff.

> She was going to sign herself out, was never coming back to this hospital or this unit. I remembered what I learned at State U. and went down to her after morning report. I sat with her and asked her what she expected from this hospitalization.

When Mrs. Storey was to be admitted, Dr. Fisher had said to the researcher, "You must talk to her. She's my best public-relations agent, though her jovial manner is all a facade." Mrs. Storey, a very obese, jolly woman, had had bony metastasis for several years following surgery breast cancer. She was able to get around with a walker and wheelchair and received chemotherapy at Dr. Fisher's office. He was admitting her for close monitoring while he changed her pain control regime, since the one she had been on was no longer effective. He started her on an oral drug, which did give her relief of pain, but one side effect of the drug was gastrointestinal upset. Mrs. Storey, despite the use of the antacid at her bedside, developed belching, nausea, and dry vomiting. She was unable to eat and was very restless, yet the drug relieved her pain to such an extent that she was able to thrash around in bed with much less pain than she had had on admission. One of the nurses had noted that the gastrointestinal symptoms started before she was started on the new medication.

Dr. Fisher was stymied. He did not want to stop the pain relief drug, but could not explain her symptoms. Karen suggested hypercalcemia but the lab tests and X-rays he ordered were unchanged from previous ones. On rounds he sat on Mrs. Storey's bed, held her hand, asked a series of questions, teased her (and she him), questioned her in detail about her symptoms. He acknowledged that he had no explanation, but he teasingly said, "Well, we'll have to order a strategy. Karen, write down, 'order a strategy.'" Eventually Dr. Fisher apologetically ordered IVs for Mrs. Storey because she was becoming dehydrated. Her eructations could be heard all the way down the hall.

Because there was no plausible explanation for her symptoms, Mrs. Storey believed that Dr. Fisher and the nurses were withholding information from her. It was hard for her to accept that Dr. Fisher truly didn't know. She told Annette that no one was explaining what was happening to her. But whatever the cause, the symptoms abated. She continued to get relief from the pain medication, and she was discharged improved. Later, she wrote to the staff with an apology:

> ... for any trouble that was caused by my actions that night and the next morning. . . . I hope I was not too far out of line (still don't quite understand it). I wish Annette was here to talk to. You are all a special breed of nurse (that is the wrong word) but may I say especially to Annette that I pray you will continue and not get discouraged by people like me. You were grand to me that morning, and I did appreciate it. I wish you could have just stayed with me until the doctor came. Sorry to keep rambling, not quite normal (?) yet. Again, thanks to all and my apologies.

Seven months later the researcher met Mrs. Storey during one of her regular visits to Dr. Fisher's office. She recognized the researcher and recalled her hospitalization experience, "You know, I was so afraid. I got worse after I went to the hospital. So many people I knew were dying, including people on my street. I was wondering, is this the end and nobody is telling me. I guess it must have gotten to me at the time."

Staff Coping Mechanisms

The staff agreed that they got along well together. Lisa said, "The staff really cares. Everyone gets involved here with their patients." Another commented, "The staff supports each other—basically we get along with each other." Still another said, "We talk over our problems, and it helps us to get over them." Annette added, "I think it's a special society. I couldn't ask for better people to work with." One staff member observed that when one person was feeling down or had a problem it affected the mood of the rest of the staff.

Karen stated:

When somebody's had a bad day around here it does get passed around a bit. The atmosphere of the day is set mostly by me. I'm not saying that because I'm the leader or something. If I come in like a grouch, everybody else will be grouchy. Whoever is in charge sets the pace for the day. If a nurse doesn't feel good, I tell her to tell the others to bug off for the day—everybody has a bad day once in a while when they don't feel up to par.

The nursing staff identified humor as their major coping mechanism. Though culture instills the idea that solemnity is the correct attitude in the presence of the very sick and dying, the staff found that laughing together was highly important to them for tension release, reassurance, disparagement of other individuals and groups in the subculture, and increased group solidarity. This was expressed in many statements. Alice said, "The people who work here have that frivolity—a sense of humor about them. That keeps us going. We look for a sense of humor in a new nurse."

Marlene added, "Laughter gives us a lift in our hearts," and Libby said, "Everyone on this floor has a sense of humor. There's always something funny." Everybody at the nurses' station laughed one day when Karen returned from rounds with Dr. Fisher and said that Mr. MacDougall told them that some old lady (Libby MacGregor) nearly dropped him on the floor three times.

Annette said:

We laugh a lot. We have been in the cafeteria reminiscing about incidents, about silly things, and laughing so loudly that everyone is looking in our direction. They are silly things, like someone almost got dropped out of the Hoyer lift. At the time it's almost tragic because you're concerned about the patient. But after you laugh about it, it just makes the day go that much easier.

Though humor and laughter were identified as the staff's coping mechanisms, Annette also mentioned that laughter was helpful to patients:

Now the patients in 247 have been pretty sick. But today Loretta Walters is awake and talking. Mrs. Kaiser has less pain and is more comfortable, and there's a new patient who is a dear. She's very ill, but she worries about you when you're getting her up. They're able to be a little bit humorous and that's important. A little laughter is the world's best medicine.

The staff also used humor to relieve the frustrations of the work situation. During the orientation classes, the researcher and the rest of the group were told that the Housekeeping Department cleaned the unit once a day, and any other spills or messes had to be cleaned up by the nursing staff. One day, when the researcher heard laughter in Mrs. Georgetti's room, she looked in, knowing that the patient was semicomatose. She saw Karen mopping the floor, which was wet because a bathroom sink had overflowed, and the other nurses laughing at the ridiculousness of a head nurse doing that when she had so many other responsibilities. "I often wind up with a mop. It's a big joke," Karen said. The researcher wondered how Mrs. Georgetti was reacting to the laughter, if she heard it, but she showed no response.

Sometimes laughter seemed inappropriate. For example, when the researcher was waiting to make rounds with the head nurse, Mildred came from the opposite direction, took the researcher's arm, and said, laughing, "Go into Mrs. Wiley and Mrs. Walters, they're both crying, and Mrs. Luckman is wiped out from diarrhea. Back there is a mess [still laughing]."

When the researcher and the head nurse went into Mrs. Wiley's room, Mrs. Wiley, paralyzed from midchest level, said, "Oh, what a night of Haitian voodoo I've had." She described a night of unrelieved pain in her right leg and a burning sensation in the heel. "If only someone would have picked it up for me." She said she had wanted to call her husband at home at five in the morning to tell him to come in and raise her leg for her. The researcher pulled back the covers, but there was nothing visible on Mrs. Wiley's heel, and her feet were propped against a footboard. The head nurse told the LPN to give Mrs. Wiley a range of motion exercises. This was not written in the care plan though the researcher had been present when it was discussed on rounds several days before.

Across the hall from Mrs. Wiley's room, Loretta Walters, paralyzed also, was crying, but Karen walked past her bed to Mrs. Varney's. Mrs. Luckman, the third patient in the room, said, "No one helped me to the bathroom. I had to go myself and I'm exhausted."

Mrs. Walters grabbed the researcher's arm and said, "I was on an awful trip last night. I was on an orange cloud." Crying, she said, "I'm tired of being sick. I don't want that diarrhea again." (It was explosive—all over the commode and herself the day before.) "I don't trust anybody any more. I don't believe anybody about my illness. When am I going to be better? I'm afraid of this day."

In an effort to cope with the high feeling states generated in the sub-culture, the nursing staff also used sarcasm and verbal sharing of feelings and experiences at lunch, coffee break, impromptu gatherings, and at Ted's biweekly conferences. (With vacation and other interruptions in Ted's schedule, the interval was sometimes three or four weeks.)

Ted had been requested to conduct these conferences after a former assistant director of nursing resigned; her method of staff support had been transactional analysis. Ted left the focus of the discussion up to the staff. He was always early for the conference, but as the year progressed, staff members drifted in later and later. If staff didn't start the discussion, Ted would initiate it by restating points made at the previous conference or by posing questions. "What do you do with feelings about your own deaths?" "Do you have a different view of life after working on this unit?" "What would you change if you knew you had a year to live?" were some of the questions. Staff reaction to the conferences was mixed.

Lisa commented:

In the beginning I felt verbal relief. Now we discuss the same things over and over. We don't come to any answers or problem solving. I'm getting frustrated with Ted. I expect him to change it and make it right. It's too unfocused, with no purpose any more. We were supposed to get help working out our feelings about death, but we haven't done it in an organized way. Patients help me grow the most.

In contrast, Mildred said:

I don't care for them [the conferences] at all. I'm very unhappy with them. With Gertrude Kelly we had a little course and some mind expansion and some problem-solving. We've got too much into death and dying and neglected other problems.

Vivian appreciated the conferences but said, "We need somebody on call to us all the time, not just every two weeks." New staff members cited Ted's conferences as helpful. He would usually ask new staff members if they had any frustrations or other strong emotional responses to the work of the unit. Susan, an RN who was returning to nursing after an absence of twelve years, said she felt frustrated because she didn't have the power or authority "to tell these people there is no hope." Ted tried to get the group to discuss feelings about their own deaths.

Alice said, "I wouldn't go through what Flo Dunaway and Jack Kravitz went through."

Libby contributed, "I just hope I never end up like that."

The researcher was interested in knowing if staff could leave the problems behind them when they left the work situation. Karen said, "I can leave the patients' problems behind, but I do take the staff problems home."

Mildred (who was then looking for another job) said she had an unwinding ritual. When she got home she made a cup of tea, took her dog, and went out to her garden. She added: "I don't have a husband to discuss things with. My two teenagers don't want to hear, 'Oh, I'm so tired.'" Speaking of her job search, Mildred added:

> I just don't enjoy that hectic hassle. I want an atmosphere where I can accomplish what I think has to be done. I can't do an adequate job if there are ten other stresses. There's no time, working full time here and having two teenaged children and a home, to have some fun in life.

Jill said that she was much more demanding when she got home than with her previous job. "I want to be pampered. I make more demands on my husband. I'm physically tired, and I don't like to make one extra trip upstairs."

Lisa was single, and her home situation was not a source of release for job pressures. She commented:

> At home, nobody wants to hear about drainage, openings, and death. They would be more objective and a help to me, but it's depressing to them. My moods at home change and I may be quiet for a couple of days, low, sad. I may have a dream about a patient. Half the people are on their way off this earth. Some days the abscesses or a lot of diarrhea really get to you, like when you have your period or something. Sputum bothers me.

"What helps then?" the researcher asked.

Lisa replied, "I tell myself, if this was my friend or relative it wouldn't even bother me. I've never had to switch assignments. I'm not a queasy person."

Rita did have difficulty adjusting to the unit and told the researcher:

> I can leave my work behind at the end of the day except for some fleeting thoughts about certain patients. Occasionally I have a nightmare. The pain and agony patients go through to buy time rather than cure upsets me. I'm scaring my husband with some of the tales.

Two staff members told the researcher that coping with the unit was a continuing struggle for them. Ruth stated:

> I have many ups and downs. At times it's very depressing. I've even asked for a transfer at times. As a matter of fact, even recently I've done that. It wasn't just the floor. I have five children and my husband travels during the week. I'm going to school taking a course for my RN. I go through times when I can hardly cope with the agony these families go through. There's a lot of tragedy here. I do take the problems home and that's difficult. I'm hard on myself. My husband is tired when he gets home. He says, "Let's not talk about that at dinner." My daughters have their own interests.

Vivian also found the work depressing at times. She added:

It does your heart good to help some of these people, but when you see them come back and come back and see them getting worse, it does make you depressed. I feel my efforts are just useless. But then again, I see somebody who knows he has cancer and knows he has only one reality and they're going to fight until the very last breath, then I feel good.

Like with Shelley Robinson. When she came in here she couldn't even walk. I have the greatest respect for somebody like that. She knows what she has, but she's not going to let it get her down.

But with Mrs. Varney—you know she's going to go further downhill. But she doesn't try, That depresses me; that's the type I stay away from. I'm afraid I couldn't show compassion for her. She's depending on everyone to do everything for her. I lose patience with somebody like that.

I have up days and down days. I don't think I can handle it, really. Emotion-wise I walk around sort of holding my breath to keep from letting my true emotions from showing, and I go home and take it out on my family. Just sometimes, not all the time because we do have some very good days here.

I am indeed ready for a change.

I yell and I scream at my kids [one was three and one was nine], and I'm a nervous wreck. I chew my nails continuously.

I've begun to resent that I'm taking it home to my family. You shouldn't have to pick on them because you're emotionally drained. Sometimes I hate the idea of coming in here in the morning.

Both Ruth and Vivian attempted to cope by partial withdrawal, going from a full-time, five-day work week to four days, even though this involved an economic hardship.

Individual members of the nursing staff identified successful adaptation to personal losses, the experience of the dying of close relatives, religious beliefs, and the "maturity that comes with aging" as helpful in successfully adapting to work on the Oncology Unit.

Gratification

The nursing staff did appreciate feedback that they were meeting patients' needs. As described, a number of patients and families sent thank-you letters, and some came back to visit. Jack Georgetti sent flowers after his wife died, "To the beautiful ladies of EH II. Thanks."

Mrs. De Lilla and Mrs. Smith sent a joint letter of appreciation about their nursing care as well as the medical care of Dr. Long and the support of Father Joe to the hospital administrator and the nursing staff while they were still hospitalized. Some thanks came indirectly, as when Mr. Hanley's relatives told Lisa how much he liked having her care for him. Lisa didn't know Mr. Hanley "felt like that. Even though he's confused now I still enjoy talking to him." Lisa also added that she enjoyed taking care of the sicker patients, but:

Some patients do not give gratification no matter what you do. For some patients, happiness is just not realistic, even though you do their treatments well and try to keep them happy. They never were happy, and you're not going to do anything that will make them any different, especially when circumstances are totally unfavorable.

At Christmas, Dr. Fisher sent the nursing staff one dozen roses and a thank you note for the care they gave his patients; Dr. Long donated funds for an afternoon Christmas party for the staff, and Dr. Thomas left a box of candy at the nurses' station.

Staff Suggestions for Improvement

The staff realized they were working within limitations, and they had ideas about how to improve the situation. For example, Rosa, a three-to-eleven LPN, said, "The unit should provide more opportunity for nurses to relate to patients. They need someone to talk to more than a bed pan."

All staff agreed there should be a kitchenette as well as a lounge for patients and families so they could get out of the confinement of the hospital room and meet others. Some knew that Elisabeth Kübler-Ross, a psychiatrist, had recommended a "crying room" on units where there was a high incidence of terminal illness, but they thought EH II staff needed "a laughing and crying room."

Vivian commented:

Even more than a psychiatrist, we could use a male nurse. Last week we only had four female patients and the rest were men. The men would like to relate to another male, especially the ones with prostate or bladder cancer, or lesions on the penis, like Tommy Smith [a leukemia patient]. It wasn't a venereal disease, because the tests came back negative, but he was so embarrassed. They [the other nurses] just couldn't understand where he was coming from being embarrassed. They could understand it, but they treated it as a joke. Some way, Dr. Thomas got to make rounds to Tommy alone. One day he asked me if I minded leaving.

Reality Shock

Much has been written in the nursing literature about the role transformation of the baccalaureate nursing student when she becomes a hospital employee, with the exception that she assume a leadership/change-agent role after a period of orientation in the work situation. The following situation not only illustrates problems in role transformation experienced by one of the staff nurses, but also points out some common problems on an oncology unit to which all staff members must adapt.

Annette and Donna were both new baccalaureate graduates, Annette one year earlier then Donna. Both were aides at Charles during their student days; both elected to work on the Oncology Unit. Annette, as previously noted in this study, survived in the system, and her transfer to the Inservice Education Department was unanimously viewed as a loss to the unit. Dr. Fisher sincerely regretted her transfer, saying Annette had "a blend of intelligence and compassion," and, "We need college graduates on this unit." Donna did not survive. What were the differences?

Annette described her adjustment to the unit:

> It's a shock to see so many ill people at one time and especially so many terminally ill. If I wasn't prepared by working on EH II the summers I worked, I would have had a more difficult time adjusting. I did have an adjustment period as an RN with new roles and responsibilities, but at least I knew the type of patient here.

During her student days, Donna was a "floating aide," that is, she was assigned to any unit in the hospital that needed an aide, so she could move in and out of situations without too much involvement. During her orientation period to EH II as a graduate nurse, she was seemingly able to assume the role responsibilities of a team member. However, the added stress of the team leadership role uncovered a major adaptational problem. One day, two months after she started working on the unit, Donna became "hysterical" after a patient, with whom she had developed a close relationship, hemorrhaged and died unexpectedly.

Karen had noted inadequacies in Donna's performance as team leader. She observed that Donna would walk past a patient in obvious discomfort and not stop to help. Donna noted some inadequacies in her own role performance. For example, one day, when Mildred returned to work after a three-day absence, she went to the desk to tell Karen about Mrs. Zelda, a patient receiving radiation therapy for spinal metastasis.

> That poor woman—what she's been through. She's paralyzed; she's worrying about money. At Plains Hospital they ordered a psychiatric consult to find out why she was depressed. She asked the psychiatrist, "If you were paralyzed from the neck down, wouldn't you be depressed?" "You don't need me," he replied, "you need a medical doctor." She needs a social-service consultation, a physical therapy consultation, and to be put on the bowel program.

When Donna heard this, she looked through the patient's chart and said to the researcher, "I can't ever do that."

"Do what?" asked the researcher.

Donna replied, "Like I had this lady the past three days. I thought I did a full assessment, but I didn't pick up the social service referral, the bowel program, or P. T." The researcher later looked at Mrs. Zelda's nursing care plan and found it blank.

After the hysteria episode, the director and the assistant director of nursing, the supervisor, and the head nurse held a conference. The supervisor and assistant director thought Donna should be transferred off the unit immediately. The head nurse thought that perhaps Donna had been given too much responsibility too soon and that they should withdraw her team leadership responsibilities temporarily and let her resume them gradually. The director of nursing agreed. The supervisor attributed Donna's problem to the particular nursing program she attended. She said:

It's quite different from the one Annette went to. They don't get the clinical experience. She hasn't come in contact with life. She didn't know how to organize her work—just didn't know where to begin. She hadn't had a pharmacology course and had to learn meds from the bottom up. I know she's very idealistic. She can't take the idealism of a baccalaureate setting and reconcile it with the real world; but lots of nurses do and I'm sure it's traumatic for them in the beginning to find out that things aren't the way they're supposed to be at all, but that's the world and that's the way it is.

Initially the head nurse was optimistic. She observed that Donna "didn't do her share of the workload. She couldn't stand really sick people." But Karen thought that if Donna's self-confidence could be gradually built up, "we will all have a part in getting her over this bad time."

The researcher talked with Donna, who said:

I chose this unit because I saw good nursing care here. But I guess I made a mistake. It's all too intense. There's too much to do. Those three men in 285 with lung cancer, they constantly spit up mucus. By two o'clock, I'm grossed out. I thought I could help here. My bag is the heart and the mind.

The researcher clarified, "You mean providing emotional support to patients?"

"Yes," Donna said.

"That's so needed here," the researcher commented.

"But," said Donna pleadingly, *"I can't get past the mucus and the shit."*

The plan was to relieve Donna of team leader responsibilities and gradually increase her patient assignment as a team member. Donna said she was relieved not to be team leader, adding, "I really don't like telling people what to do. When I'm team leader and in charge of others, I find I overlook things which should not be overlooked on this floor." But Donna continued to have difficulty with planning and completing nursing care. She told the researcher:

It just seems like this floor is so intense. There's so much to think about. Constipation, impactions, and diarrhea are such a problem. On the other floors if you don't ask a patient if he wants his back rubbed, if you forget, it's no big deal. But here, their skin breaks down. I finally got over the hurdle to do mouth care routinely every day. It wasn't difficult to do, but it was just something that wasn't embedded into my routine and it's something you just can't overlook here because of the mouth lesions. It's just really, really intense.

In addition to the intensity of the nursing care, Donna had a major problem coping with death and relating to dying patients. "It hit me," she said, "two months into being here when the lady in 245 died. I really went to pieces." In nursing school Donna had been able to evade this issue. She said:

Like at school we discussed death and dying from the time I got there. But I haven't related Kübler-Ross to my emotions yet, so I haven't developed any coping mechanisms yet. In my Med-Surg experience I had a patient with bronchogenic carcinoma. I knew I was supposed to put down in my care plan things like reassurance, deal with the fact that he was dying, but I really couldn't handle that. At conference we talked about it. A lot of kids got into laughing about parents and friends dying, but I was silent. I just didn't want it to enter my mind. I guess that's my defense mechanism—denial—blocking it out, or I'll cross that bridge when I come to it type thing.

Donna was perturbed that the staff thought she'd "lived life in a gilded cage, shallow, inexperienced. In fact, Mrs. MacGregor has told me that." Donna told the researcher that she'd worked since she was thirteen years old and, "I've never had anything given to me." She also acknowledged that she had never experienced a personal loss. No pets or close members of the family died; only a grandmother she never knew. When the researcher was discussing this with Donna, she said:

I don't like to think about that. I prefer not to think about it. I'm so much into being alive, easy come, easy go. Take today, not tomorrow. I enjoy life so much that I don't even like to think about that. But now here I am thinking about it, but it's still distant, not anything close. When my mother talks to me about the possibilty of my father's death, I can't tolerate it. I think it's terrible.

Some staff members resented the fact that Donna, who had received her RN licensure, was not carrying her fair share of the workload. Others were more concerned about her growth. Jill, the aide, said, "Donna is uptight. She can't laugh and she needs to. I've seen her crying with some patients who are dying. I've had to sit with her and she says, 'Talk to me, talk to me.'"

Annette, who observed Donna go into the dying Mrs. Harris's room four different times just to watch her for ten to fifteen minutes, thought Donna was trying to accept the fact that Mrs. Harris was dying. "Mrs. Harris was a positive stroker," Annette said, "and Donna thought she was a really classy person. But when she started to go downhill and was unable to give strokes, Donna asked not to be assigned to her any more.'' Annette thought Donna was going through the grieving process. "I'm glad at least that she went back. She could have avoided that, too," said Annette.

Donna later told the researcher that she had decided to go into Mrs. Harris' room when she was close to death to offer some support to her husband, who was sitting at the bedside. "But I was the one who fell apart," she said, adding, "When I started crying, he just turned his head away."

Donna readily acknowledged that she formed closer attachments with some patients than with others. She described herself as an affectionate person who invested a great deal of herself in everything she did. "The day I see Mrs. Menna come in flat on her back is the day I'm leaving the floor. The day Mr. Snead goes (dies) is the day I go, really," said Donna.

The head nurse and supervisor agreed that when, after several weeks, Donna was again given the full role responsibilities of team leader, she did not show evidence of growth. Avoidance behavior, such as going to early coffee break and prolonging it and sometimes not starting her patient care assignments until close to noon, was common. Her attitude of denigrating certain job functions was difficult for the supervisor to take. Frances related one part of a conversation with Donna, who said:

> For four years all they ever stressed [in school] was what was going on in a patient's head. Now you're expecting me to be concerned about whether or not I've signed off a drug or all kinds of administrative nitty-gritty-type things that we have to do. For four years what was important was how a person felt and reacted. Frankly, I couldn't care whether I sign off that drug today or tomorrow. I don't think that's important. What's important is that I gave it.

Donna did not seem to appreciate the fact that by not signing off a drug as given, she was exposing the patient to the harm of a possible second dose by an unsuspecting nurse.

The supervisor's appraisal of Donna after she resumed team leader functions was that she continued to do poorly, including involvement in medication errors. She was placed on thirty-days probation because of her overall performance evaluation. Finally, after six months of experience on EH II, the supervisor said,

> We prayed Donna out. She never developed any more insight. She was never given full responsibility the last month of employment. She was uncomfortable giving medications. She's gone to a university hospital to work on a primary care nursing unit. I'd be interested in knowing how she does. Her letter of resignation was strange. I think she needed more counseling than any one of us was prepared to give.

In the primary nursing care system, a nurse is assigned to a patient on admission and is responsible for his or her nursing care for the duration of hospitalization and for readmissions. This system decentralizes authority and emphasizes accountability and autonomy of the professional nurse working with a group of patients. Movement toward an all RN staff is a natural outcome of such a system. The researcher asked Annette what she thought of the primary nursing model for EH II. She commented, "I have a question whether primary nursing would work on a unit like this. Part of the problem is that the patients are here so long—can a nurse take it? Even the lifting and moving would be a hazard. With the real problem patients they need a switch after a week."

EPILOGUE

In a conversation three months after field data collection ended, the head nurse seemed optimistic. Two full-time staff nurses, a male aide, and a ward clerk had been hired for the day shift. Dr. Long had donated some casual furniture and art reproductions to the unit to create a lounge area at one end of the corridor so that patients could get out of their rooms. He also acquired a female physician associate who was well received by the staff. He had agreed to meet with them to discuss his philosophy of treatment, but stipulated that for each individual patient they wanted to question him about, they would have to pose an alternate treatment solution.

Dr. Thomas had provided funds for Karen and a staff nurse to attend a continuing education course in oncology nursing given by a nearby university. One of Karen's course goals was to obtain materials that could be developed into an orientation program for the EH II staff.

The researcher's visits to the Oncology Unit ended after fifteen months. Of the EH II staff she met from three shifts, all but one was working because of economic necessity. Most were primary home managers as well. In addition to the demanding nature of the work on the Oncology Unit in both expressive and instrumental aspects, all had personal and family concerns reflective of life in an era of rapid change. During the period of the study, one individual was fired; one left to seek new growth experiences; one became the primary breadwinner because of her husband's chronic illness; one left for another department; one failed to adapt to the subculture and left; one left after failing the state RN licensing examination twice; one's twenty-three-year-old son was killed in an automobile accident; one had a baby girl; one retired; one left for further education; one took a leave of absence after her mother had surgery for cancer and her husband had a shunt for renal dialysis (she returned to work on the night shift); one moved from the area; one male LPN on the night shift early in the study year transferred to the emergency room; three went from full time to four days a week; one got married; and, after a long series of thefts of money and personal belongings from patients, one was entrapped and dismissed, refusing an offer of psychiatric help.

Chapter 6
Patients and Families

Data on patients and families have been inextricably woven into the previous chapters. This chapter provides some general information about the patients and their support systems and also addresses specific problems experienced by patients, families, and staff.

PATIENTS

Statistics

Charles Hospital had no central source from which data on admissions, discharges, and deaths could be retrieved. The researcher obtained some information from a fiscal officer; she compiled the data on deaths by reviewing one year's records in the Admissions Office. In the twelve months of the research there were 358 direct admissions to EH II. This number included individuals with more than one admission, but did not include admissions to EH II by transfer from other units. The number of discharges recorded was 407. The average length of stay for patients on EH II was 24.1 days, compared with 11.2 days for the rest of the hospital.

During the year, 91 patients died, approximately one out of every four to five patients admitted. On the day shift, 38 patients died; on the evening shift, 29; and during the night, 24.

No record of place of residence was kept for EH II patients. For the hospital as a whole, 36 percent were from the city of Lafayette. No person whom the researcher questioned, including Dr. Fisher and the supervisor, knew what route existed for Charles' clinic patients, basically, the inner-city poor, to receive specialized cancer care, either inpatient or outpatient. It was thought that clinic patients were probably treated on the general medical or gynecologic services unless they were considered unusual cases and were referred to an oncologist. Dr. Fisher said he would be glad to treat Medicare or Medicaid patients who could get to his suburban office; however, it was not accessible by public transportation.

Charles Hospital had no tumor registry; therefore, there were no available statistics regarding the primary tumor sites of patients admitted to EH II; nor were follow-up data available. It was the researcher's impression that the primary site of cancer for the majority of male patients was the lung, and for females, the breast, which would coincide with national figures on disease incidence.

Early Detection

The comments of many patients pointed out the importance of addressing the affective component of educational programs for prevention or early detection of cancer. For example, Mrs. De Lilla and Mrs. Burnham were roommates. Mrs. De Lilla had multiple metastatic sites from breast cancer, but these had been controlled for some time. At one point, she was admitted for treatment of pneumonia and received oxygen intermittently from a cylinder at her bedside. Mrs. De Lilla objected to her roommate smoking in the room, so Mrs. Burnham grudgingly sat out in the hallway whenever she wanted to smoke. Mrs. Burnham, who was receiving radiation therapy for lung cancer, had been advised by Dr. Long not to smoke, but her reply to him was, "Listen, half of the patients downstairs [in the Radiation Therapy Department] have lung cancer, and they all smoke while they're waiting."

Mrs. De Lilla's comment to Dr. Long about her roommate was, "She's a hard number. The nurses are compassionate, but the patients aren't."

The researcher casually remarked to Sharon, one of the LPNs, that she was appalled at the toll taken by breast cancer, that apparently the early detection education programs were not reaching a great many women. Sharon agreed and remarked, "Look at Mrs. Caffery. She was admitted for a decompressive laminectomy for spinal metastasis, which left her unable to walk. But her primary tumor was never diagnosed. She has a breast tumor which is a huge, draining mass."

The patient, Mrs. Caffery, said to Alice, "They said I have a what-do-you-call-it. I don't want to know about it, but I do want them to do what they have to do."

Later Alice saw another patient with breast cancer talking with Mrs. Caffery. Alice remarked:

> I don't usually see patients in talking to Mrs. Caffery, but she hasn't had any family in to visit her. Sometimes patients help each other. She doesn't want to know the true facts. I know her doctor told her, but he wrote on her chart that she "doesn't want to know."

Follow-Up

Individual nurses were heard asking doctors, the social worker, the public health coordinator, or Midge, Dr. Fisher's office nurse, for follow-up information on discharged patients to satisfy their own interest or curiosity. The obituary columns of local newspapers were another source of information, which the older staff members, Libby and Alice, usually reported on. Sometimes obituaries were posted at the nurses' station. Occasionally a discharged patient would come back to visit.

The researcher had observed Mr. Louis being simulated for spinal radiation in the Radiation Therapy Department, so when he strode with sprightly step onto the unit one day, she recognized him. He checked to see who was behind the desk at the nurses' station, then quietly slipped a gold piece into Mildred's and Karen's hands, surprising them. He said he had come to the hospital that day for lab tests and added, "When I was first admitted I couldn't walk across the street, and now I can walk for miles." He also asked about Rosa, the evening-shift LPN who had been pregnant at the time of his hospitalization. (She had had a baby girl two days after her due date.)

Age

The age of patients ranged from sixteen (three girls) to ninety-one (Mrs. Stone). The three youngest were Margie Jackson, who had malignant lymphoma but was admitted briefly for treatment of a transfusion reaction she had suffered as an outpatient; Laura Boxer, who was admitted from another hospital for radiation therapy following chest surgery for malignant lymphoma; and Susan Graham, who received radiation therapy for a brain tumor.

The eldest, Mrs. Stone, was transferred to Charles from a county hospital for the aged, where she had been admitted one week previously. The major problem stated on her chart by the transferring hospital was, "Patient is unable to communicate." The doctors discovered that Mrs. Stone's tongue was completely replaced by tumor. Surgeons advised against tracheostomy and tube feedings. The radiologist determined that the tumor was most likely incurable by radiation but that Mrs. Stone could benefit from palliative radiation therapy to decrease pain.

On admission, the nurses found that Mrs. Stone could speak but that she was withdrawn and suspicious. With supportive care she was able to sit in a chair and occasionally take some liquids or soft food. Since she was unable to take enough by mouth for adequate hydration, Mrs. Stone was given intravenous fluids. Gradually, she developed an oral infection and other complications and grew progressively worse. One afternoon about four weeks after Mrs. Stone's admission, the head nurse accompanied a cardiac consultant to the bedside. When Karen went to turn her for the cardiologist's examination, she realized that Mrs. Stone had died.

The staff particularly regretted the diagnosis of cancer in the young girls and in the three young men with testicular cancer. But the age group that seemed most difficult for the nursing staff, from the points of view of social loss, family stress, loss of body image, functioning, and independence, as well as pain, suffering, and anger, were those in their late thirties to early fifties. Patients in this age bracket often had young children as well as aging parents.

Forty-seven-year-old Mrs. Denise Dionne had been diagnosed as having rectal cancer when she was admitted to another hospital after hemorrhaging while volunteering at her church's summer fair. Urinary tract complications, abscesses, and fistula formation following colostomy surgery kept her hospitalized for five months before she was transferred to Charles for radiation therapy for pelvic metastasis. Mrs. Dionne admittedly came to Charles with a "chip on my shoulder" because of bitterness about her surgeon. "When I asked him questions, he hollered at me and put me down terribly. They should train doctors that patients have a right to know what's happening to themselves," she stated.

Despite Dr. Fisher's directness about her diagnosis and the chronicity of the disease, Mrs. Dionne had high hopes for cure. She told the researcher:

> I've just got to get home; I have so many responsibilities. My daughters are only fourteen and sixteen; I have a seventeen-year-old son and two older ones. My mother is semisenile in a nursing home. My husband brought her home for Christmas even though I wasn't there. It's hard on him. He comes in every night and he's managing the home and the kids, too. It's amazing how people you hardly know help you when you need it. One friend visits my mother in the nursing home once a week. You think your children grow away from you, but one of my older boys calls me every day, sometimes more than once.

A nurse from the hospital where Mrs. Dionne had had her surgery visited her at Charles once and later told the researcher that Mr. Dionne looked as if he had aged ten years in the seven and a half months of Mrs. Dionne's hospitalization. At Charles, the patient's high hopes were dashed on several occasions. Her radiation therapy had to be temporarily suspended because of skin reaction, and she had another setback when Dr. Fisher told her she should learn injection technique so that she could give herself pain medication at home. She had expected to go home pain-free. She did learn the technique, however, as well as other aspects of self-care. She died about six months after discharge.

Appearance

Unlike the frequently portrayed photographs of cancer patients, many of

EH II's patients were not progressively cachectic, though the dying ones, of course, underwent obvious physical changes. With regard to the general appearances of patients, Rita, a new staff nurse, commented, "I thought the patient's would be at death's door, I'd just be turning them over. I'm surprised that so many seem so relatively well. I was scared." Though most lost some weight in the course of treatment, many patients weighed over two hundred pounds. Alice, the aide, did not agree with many of the staff's negative view of Loretta Walters, an exceptionally heavy patient. Alice said:

> I took care of Mrs. Walters for seven days. I got along fine with her. Some people find her difficult. Some of her days *are* difficult. The difficulty with Mrs. Walters for all of us was to have to lift all 280 pounds of her onto the stretcher, which was four to six inches higher than the bed.

Loretta was discharged after ten weeks to a nursing home and was re-admitted to Charles about nine months later, very ill with peritonitis. When the researcher mentioned to the head nurse that Mrs. Walters was a patient on another unit, Karen remarked, "The nurses' backs are just about recovering from her last visit."

Many of the women lost their hair as a result of chemotherapy and wore wigs that gave them a well-groomed appearance. (Some men became bald but didn't look too unusual). But Mrs. Knull's daughter was found crying in the hall when her mother was admitted; the daughter was upset because she thought her mother was sharing a room with a male patient, but the patient was Mrs. Austin, who was too sick to care about wearing her wig, and her baldness and steroid-induced Cushing's syndrome gave her a masculine appearance. A few women developed a deep, bronze skin color.

Some of the patients looked very healthy. Once during afternoon report in the conference room, Mr. Todt, who had had triple chemotherapy by vein in the morning, walked by, dressed in street clothes. He backed up and said good-by to the group, telling them he was discharged. Donna asked who was taking him home.

"You're looking at him," he said.

"You mean you're driving yourself home?" asked Donna.

"Why not, there's nothing wrong with me," he commented. He walked away, then backed up again and said, "Nothing wrong with me except cancer, that's all." He had Hodgkin's disease.

Mr. Vandeveer, a trim, athletic-looking man in his mid-forties, was ambulatory and did walk around the ward. He had been transferred from a nearby hospital where he had been scheduled for routine surgery for a hernia repair. At surgery, the "hernia" was found to be a malignant lymphoma. His daughter, an RN and former staff nurse at Charles, selected Dr. Fisher to treat her father. She came in on the evening shift to be her father's private-duty nurse. Mr. Vandeveer was highly anxious because of the suddenness of the diagnosis and the fact that the surgeon had not removed the entire tumor. Dr. Fisher asked the nurses to ask Mr. Vandeveer's daughter, Maggie, not to wear her nurse's uniform when she came in to take care of her father; he thought that this concentrated nursing attention was leading Mr. Vandeveer to believe he was sicker than any one else on the unit. He had developed a wound infection that delayed the start of his radiation therapy. The wound was incised and drained and packed with sterile gauze.

On rounds, Mr. Vandeveer said to Dr. Fisher, "Couldn't I have a pair of tweezers to pull some of this packing out?"

"No, replied Dr. Fisher.

"Maybe some of the stuff will come out with it," said Mr. Vandeveer.

"No," repeated Dr. Fisher.

"Couldn't that be growing in there? Why the hell didn't he take it all out?" asked Mr. Vandeveer.

Dr. Fisher replied, "The tumor was close to arteries and veins and a major nerve to your leg. Since you were going to get radiation and chemotherapy anyway, it wasn't worth risking a major complication." Dr. Fisher increased the dosage of Mr. Vandeveer's tranquilizer. Further tests showed bone marrow involvement. Mr. Vandeveer completed his course of radiation therapy and was started on chemotherapy. A year later, Maggie said her father was working and was asymptomatic, though still receiving chemotherapy.

Physiologic Problems

Common physiologic problems experienced by patients included pain, undernutrition, anemia, and leukopenia with consequent susceptibility to infection, mouth lesions, and skin breakdown. Blood transfusions were ordered to keep blood elements at a therapeutic level and to replace blood in patients with active bleeding. Esophagitis, anorexia, nausea, vomiting, or diarrhea were not uncommon side effects of systemic chemotherapy or radiation therapy to the chest or abdominal area. Control of these symptoms was attempted with medication and supportive nursing care. Occasionally, intravenous therapy was necessary for hydration and electrolyte balance.

Narcotic drugs, bed rest, and change in diet pattern contributed to constipation, which was a frequent complaint of patients. Bed rest also contributed to the development of decubitus ulcers, thrombophlebitis, debilitation from muscle disuse, and joint contractures. More specific problems, such as pathologic fractures, intestinal obstruction, lung infection, bleeding tendencies, and states of confusion brought about by liver failure or oxygen lack from a variety of causes, were related to advancing disease.

Both patients and staff were frightened at times by patients with organic psychoses from the effects of brain tumor or with deranged metabolic states. Mr. Morgan threatened to sign himself out unless his room was changed, because his roommate kept climbing into bed with him in the middle of the night. After the roommate was thwarted in this activity, he visited the three ladies in the next room, nude. Dr. Thomas commented, "It's probably the most exciting thing that's happened to them here." But the women were quite upset.

Emotional Problems

All of the above-mentioned physiologic problems could be present and compounded in patients with spinal cord or nerve root compression from tumor involvement. Their neuromuscular deficits ranged from gait or bladder and bowel disturbances to total paralysis and loss of function below the point of spinal cord involvement. Total loss of independence proved to be the greatest difficulty for patients and families to cope with, and these patients provided the greatest nursing challenge. Even small losses of independence meant a great deal to patients. For example, Mr. Sosin, a seventy-two-year-old traveling salesman, was ready to be discharged. He had been admitted with seizures from brain metastasis, but he had responded well to radiation therapy and medication. On rounds he asked Dr. Fisher if he could continue to drive. Dr. Fisher gave an emphatic "no," leaving no room for negotiation.

"That takes everything out of me," Mr. Sosin said. He persisted in trying to get Dr. Fisher to change his mind.

Becoming increasingly annoyed, Dr. Fisher said, "We'll discuss it further when you come to the office for your follow-up visit."

One day the researcher went into a room to talk with a patient she knew, who she found sleeping. A recently admitted patient, whom the researcher did not know, was in the opposite bed. The anxiety provoked by the threat of loss of independence was poignantly described by this forty-five-year-old woman, who had accomplished and reset short-term goals a number of times after her initial cancer diagnosis. After the researcher introduced herself and explained the study, but before she could ask a single question, Valerie Whelan said, "It's the fear, the fear."

"The fear of what?" the researcher asked.

"The fear of being totally dependent. No one should be afraid to die. You just hope people you love will be able to cope with the separation, and when you find out they can, it gets you—right here [pointing to her heart]. But it's the dependence that you don't want."

In explaining how she had been admitted, Valerie said that she had surgery for breast cancer four and one-half years previously, adding, "In between seven hospitalizations I've lived an essentially normal life." Her other admissions had been for additional surgical procedures (bilateral oophorectomy and adrenalectomy), chemotherapy, and radiation therapy to various sites. She explained that she had been to Dr. Fisher's office for chemotherapy two days before this admission, then added:

> I was sitting at the breakfast table yesterday after my husband left for work and felt such sharp pain in my chest that I knew I was paralyzed. I knew I had to get to the phone, but I couldn't walk. Funny what comes to your mind at a time like that. All I could think of was "The Little Engine That Could." I've got to make it, I've got to make it, I kept saying to myself. I called Dr. Fisher and then called my sister to take me to the hospital. I believed the worst had happened, I was paralyzed. It wasn't until I was here awhile that I could believe what one of the nurses pointed out—that I had walked from the wheelchair to the bed. And my sister reminded me I had walked from the house to the car. It's the fear that gets to you.

> I vomited after chemotherapy and must have snapped a hot spot on a rib. I'm to get radiation there now. Dr. Fisher tells you what's wrong—he pulls no punches—but he tells you in an understanding way.

Father Joe visited all the patients on the Oncology Unit daily, usually in the late afternoon. He explained that while he provided for the religious needs of some patients, his major role on the unit was probably that of a friendly listener. He said:

> I try to serve more as a sponge to help patients pour out their feelings. Sometimes they can express anger and frustration to me that they can't throw out at anybody else. It's frightening to have to depend on somebody else for your most basic needs. This total dependency is the greatest source of depression I see. It must be awful not to be able to even pour a glass of water for yourself.

As has been described, the responses of patients at various stages of illness included denial, anger, depression, and acceptance. The nursing staff considered the anger of patients and families directed at them as one of the most difficult aspects of care.

During the research year, the staff noted that two patients of Dr. Long had had psychiatric consultations. The difference in approach of the two psychiatrists was notable. One patient, Loretta Walters, was labeled by the consultant as "chronic schizophrenic," and a medication was recommended. However, the psychiatrist made no suggestions regarding supportive medical care or nursing approaches that would be helpful for this woman, who also had multiple physiologic problems.

The other patient, Mr. Cunningham, had advanced lung cancer and severe constipation. He was described by Dr. Long as being severely depressed, with death ideation. The doctor wrote, "Says he wants to die, and may do it." After the night nurses reported that he was agitated and crying, Dr. Long kept him heavily sedated. On the chart Dr. Long indicated that the patient had an acute psychosis, although no behavioral description was recorded. The consultant psychiatrist described Mr. Cunningham as "not psychotic but depressed, frightened, and confused." His recommended approach was to talk with Mrs. Cunningham and their daughter to help them adjust to the patient's terminal condition without premature rejection; to decrease the amount of sedating and tranquilizing drugs, which increased his depression; to mobilize him by getting him up in a chair out in the hall; and to tolerate some agitation. Mr. Cunningham improved briefly on this regimen, but a series of thrombotic and embolic episodes culminated in his death ten days later.

FAMILIES

Family relationships ran along a continuum from loving and supportive to overtly hostile, with open bickering at the bedside. As a new aide, Jill quickly noted some of the difficult family situations.

> Two out of three in 216—their husbands are so rough. Mr. Kaiser and Mr. Edwards are doing the opposite of what the patients need. Mr. Edwards is bullying and belittling. Mrs. Edwards is like a child, she needs attention. Her husband could help by trying to read to her or to be here more often. He says things like, "How stupid you are," or, to us, "She's so dumb," and winks like that's supposed to be funny. He makes her cry. She's having physical therapy after having her pathologic fracture pinned. He says she's "like a baby, why does she have to learn to walk all over again?"

Mr. and Mrs. Schapp argued so loudly every night that they disturbed the other patients. Mrs. Schapp's frequent telephone arguments so upset her roommate, Marge Holland, that she resorted to keeping the curtain pulled, which increased Marge's own isolation. Dr. Fisher warned Mrs. Schapp that he would have to transfer her off the unit if her arguments with her husband continued to disturb other patients. Finally, one evening Mr. Schapp stormed off the unit, saying he was never coming back. A few days later, the couple were reconciled and made plans to go on a second honeymoon.

Vivian gave this view of family relationships:

> Some families are beautiful, but some are pretty disrupted. They start to bicker, then they start to keep away. I guess they do this to hold onto their sanity, but it's the worst thing for the patient. Some patients are so cantankerous you can understand why the families stay away.

Mrs. Varney had been ready to go home for three weeks, but no one would come for her. "My sons would never send me to a nursing home," she declared. But the staff and the social worker felt that none of her four sons really wanted to take responsibility for her. Though they sometimes visited in the evening, they did not respond to requests by the staff and social worker to discuss plans. Each time plans were made for Mrs. Varney's discharge, something happened. For example, she planned to stay with her son George, whose wife had just had a baby. On the day of discharge George called and said he couldn't take his mother home because his wife had moved out of the house the day before, taking the baby and the furniture with her. Two other times Mrs. Varney was set to be discharged, but she developed complications that necessitated a longer stay.

Finally one divorced son and his girlfriend said they would take care of Mrs. Varney in her own home if the fourth son would move out so they could move in. While the house was being readied, the girlfriend came in to EH II and was taught by the nurses to give Mrs. Varney the necessary physical care and injections as well as how to get her up in a chair and back to bed. Discharge day finally came, but the difficulties continued at home. The social worker got several crisis calls from both the son and his girlfriend, each accusing the other of taking Mrs. Varney's narcotics. About a month after discharge, the couple split up, and Mrs. Varney was admitted to a nursing home.

Nurses occasionally expressed the opinion to the researcher that Dr. Fisher discharged his patients too soon and that families were not ready to cope with the responsibilities. For example, Mrs. Stabile, in her late sixties, had cancer of the ovary with abdominal metastasis. She was admitted with a partial intestinal obstruction, which was treated conservatively. When she was able to retain soft food, Dr. Fisher told her and the three elderly members of her family at her bedside that she could go home. Seeing their alarmed expressions, he said, "I'm only a phone call away. Call me at any time. If you have any doubts or can't reach me immediately, call an ambulance and take her to the emergency room." Not reassured, Mrs. Stabile's husband and sister followed Dr. Fisher into the hall, saying they did not think she was ready to go home. Her bedroom was upstairs, and she didn't have the strength to go up and down. Dr. Fisher told them the visiting nurse would be in to see Mrs. Stabile daily starting the day after discharge, and the American Cancer Society would provide a bed for downstairs. Again he told them, "Call me any time."

Later, when Dr. Fisher examined Mrs. Stabile's abdomen, which was hard and distended, his facial expression changed and he tempered his optimistic attitude. He told Mrs. Stabile that he would order one more X-ray and asked if the surgeons had seen her yet. When she replied affirmatively, Dr. Fisher said, "Well, we'll see what they have to say," and added, "The biggest thing I fear about your going home is your own fear."

Out in the hall, Dr. Fisher explained to the nurses that cancer of the ovary is easy to treat if it's detected early because it tends to stay localized; but if detected late, as in Mrs. Stabile's case, it spreads "all over the abdomen." Dr. Fisher stated that the surgeons would probably recommend a colostomy. "But I'm afraid if she has surgery with her other problems [congestive heart failure] she'll never leave the hospital—a colostomy is not an easy thing to adjust to." He went on to explain that since Mrs. Stabile had multiple metastasic sites, she could even have further proximal obstruction after the colostomy was performed. He added:

I'd rather send her home, even for a few days; if she gets into trouble at home we would bring her in right away and she could have surgery within forty-eight hours. But I'm troubled about sending her home because she's from a family of old people; I've never met anyone from the family who isn't around her age.

Mrs. Stabile was discharged the following day.

Small losses sometimes compounded the large tragedies. One morning, an elderly woman, the wife of a patient, came to the nurses' station after having left the unit for twenty minutes for a cup of tea. She had left six dollars in her husband's bedside drawer in case the barber came, but the barber had not come, and the money was gone. Both patients in the room were bedridden. During that twenty minutes someone on the unit had taken money from a sick man. Who was it? The woman shrugged her shoulders and walked back to her husband.

Another patient, Mr. Plante, had lung cancer. Early in his hospitalization his family had complained because his lab tests had had to be rescheduled—he had been given two bottles of ginger ale during the night when he was supposed to be fasting. In the researcher's opinion this could easily happen, because there were no indicators at the bedside that a patient was to fast during the night.

When it was time for Mr. Plante's discharge, his wife and daughter expressed a great deal of concern to the staff because he required intramuscular injections for pain relief, and his wife was unable to master the technique to give them at home. His daughter learned the technique, but she did not live with her parents. When the staff told Dr. Fisher about this, he gave Mr. Plante a prescription for an oral narcotic. Mr. Plante told Dr. Fisher that he did not think pills would relieve his pain, but despite his and the family's concern, he was discharged. Though Mr. Plante had nausea, dyspnea, and pain during his hospitalization for lung cancer, he kept himself occupied by weaving place mats, which he sold to staff and visitors as fast as he could make them.

Eighty-year-old Mr. Ralph ambled up to the desk one day for a discharge slip and his prescriptions. He sat in a chair in the hall while the head nurse called Dr. Long's office for an appointment for him. He had been admitted for treatment of pneumonia, but staff knew him from an earlier admission for radiation therapy for cancer of the mandible. Mr. Ralph said, "I don't know whether I'm better off here or home." The wide range of family structures was evidenced by his description of his circumstances. He explained that he lived with his sisters; who were ninety and eighty-six. Both were healthy and active and, according to their brother, managed the household without additional help. He expressed some concern about how long this situation could continue.

Nurses recognized that some family members coped with the strain by unloading their emotions in angry outbursts at the nursing staff. In the conference room one afternoon, the researcher heard an hysterical commotion at the nurses' station. It was Mrs. Lorain's daughter, who had gone to her mother's bed and found it empty. Mrs. Lorain had been taken to surgery for a nerve block for pain relief. "Why did you let her go?" shouted the daughter at the head nurse, adding, "She had this change in her will to take care of."

Karen explained that Mrs. Lorain had not been scheduled for the procedure at a particular time but was to be called when the surgeon completed his scheduled cases. The transporters had come for her unexpectedly. The head nurse also explained that the procedure did not require anesthesia, then Karen took the daughter into the conference room and sat with her until she was calmer. Mrs. Lorain, in her late fifties, was hospitalized for four and one-half months for metastatic breast cancer and a pathologic fracture of the femur. She developed a huge decubitus ulcer over her sacrum which was not amenable to grafting. Her medical insurance ran out, but Dr. Long continued to treat her. Her insurance did cover around-the-clock nursing care at home, and about seven weeks after discharge, Mrs. Lorain died at home. Dr. Long had wanted to readmit her for blood transfusions, because, he said, her low hemoglobin was responsible for the weakness, tissue breakdown, and lassitude she experienced at home. However, her family refused to have her readmitted.

Seventy-year-old Mrs. Whiting was admitted with markedly advanced cancer of the rectum. She had been under medical care for some time because of thyroid and cardiovascular disease, as well as vision and hearing loss. Because of her multiple medical problems, she was considered a poor surgical risk and was being treated with radiation therapy. Dr. Fisher described Mrs. Whiting's daughter as "near hysteria," saying she called him at least three times a day. The daughter also complained that her mother was not getting enough nursing supervision. The nursing staff believed this complaint was unjustified, and they resented the daughter's behavior. For example, she thought that the disposable pads used to absorb rectal drainage were causing her mother to sweat, so she pulled out the pads and threw them on the floor. This difficult behavior continued until the mother was discharged.

Family Support

Recognizing the tremendous strains felt by families of cancer patients, the hospital established a family conference group two years after the unit was opened. The group included the social worker, the public health nursing coordinator, a chaplain, and the nursing supervisor. No physicians or members of the nursing staff of EH II participated, since it was believed that their presence might inhibit a full discussion of problems, some of which might concern a doctor or the nursing staff. A meeting was scheduled once a week after evening visiting hours, but attendance by families was poor. Staff thought this was because families did not want to leave the inner city after visiting hours, so the conference time was changed to two in the afternoon.

The researcher attended several conferences and observed that some family members were helped by the opportunity to meet and share feelings with other families. Some asked for help with specific problems. For example, a father asked for suggestions regarding the adult supervision his eleven-year-old daughter should have after his wife's death, while he was at work. One woman frankly stated that she was unable to care for her husband at home, though this was Dr. Fisher's plan. She was helped to communicate with Dr. Fisher, and the man was transferred to a community hospital closer to their home. Family members who had been to one or more conferences sometimes brought a newcomer they had met on the unit.

In a comfortable, living-room setting on the floor below the Oncology Unit, this group afforded an opportunity for professionals and family members to get to know each other much better than the limited structural arrangements for visiting on the Oncology Unit allowed. Father Joe said that occasionally a family member who attended a conference would get in touch with him after a patient died, mostly to express guilt feelings regarding whether the patient should have gone through so much suffering before death. He said that relatives tended to forget that in many cases the patient had had five or six years of relatively normal life under treatment.

A small sign on the doorway to EH II announced the time of family conference, but the major mechanism by which they were announced was through personal invitation by the head nurse or one of the staff nurses when families came to visit. Several times in November, the researcher arrived for family conference and found no families there. The next week the researcher stopped at the nurses' station and asked the supervisor if family conference was to be held as scheduled.

Frances replied, "Not that I know of; you can go down and I'll follow."

Karen added, "There isn't any family conference. Since Lisa and Annette left, we've been so busy that we haven't had time to invite the families." Thus, one of the most positive means of family and patient support went out of existence because of the nursing staff shortage and because no member of the group took the initiative to assume a leadership role and find a different mechanism for inviting families.

Family Gratitude

Mr. Piel had had cancer for six years and had experienced and recovered from several crises. This time he was on the ward for almost twelve weeks and was dying. His family spent long hours at his bedside, and his wife and sister attended the family conference when the researcher was present for the first time. Mrs. Piel said:

> Mr. Piel is asleep again. [She seemed disappointed.] Last night he was asleep when we left at eight o'clock. He slept the whole time we were there. I was wishing he'd wake up, since he was sweaty and we wanted to change him, but the nurse did call us and tell us he woke up at twenty to nine, had something to drink, was changed and comfortable.

As close as their relationship was, Mrs. Piel related there was some "mutual pretense" going on between her husband and herself. Many years before, they had put a down payment on a cemetery plot. Recently Mr. Piel, in his wife's absence, had asked his brother-in-law to go and pay off the remaining cost of the grave. The brother-in-law told Mrs. Piel, and the two of them went together. The brother-in-law told Mr. Piel that he had carried out his request but didn't tell him that Mrs. Piel had gone with him.

About a week later, on rounds with Dr. Long, Mr. Piel was noted to be pale, pasty looking, and semicomatose, but moaning with pain from several pathologic fractures. Dr. Long told Annette to increase Mr. Piel's morphine to 60 mg every two hours. Annette looked at Dr. Long and repeated the dose, and Dr. Long confirmed it. Later, when the researcher discussed the situation with Annette, she said:

> In our pharmacology course in nursing school [a baccalaureate program] we were taught that 15 mg was the maximum dose of morphine to be given at one time. I know he's been on a gradually increasing dose, but I still remember that earlier learning.

"Was the medication given as ordered?" the researcher asked.

> Oh, yes. He had two doses. Ellen [a graduate nurse] was really hesitant about giving the third. But Mr. Piel died before that was necessary. His family was with him. As they were leaving after he died, they left a beautiful letter for the nursing staff with a large sum of money to buy something for the unit. But they stressed that they didn't want to know how it was spent. It was like they didn't want to have any further connection with the unit.

Frances, the supervisor, was off that day. As Annette was reading the letter to the staff at the nurses' station, a substitute supervisor came by. Several of the staff were teary-eyed, and Annette was having a hard time getting through the reading without weeping. The substitute supervisor scolded them for getting overinvolved with the patients.

The researcher asked the head nurse if the staff were ever expected to administer a seemingly lethal dose of a drug to a terminally ill patient. "No," Karen said emphatically, adding, "That would be euthanasia. It's true some of them get high doses of narcotics, but they've been increased gradually. Pain is evaluated daily on doctors' rounds."

Families did derive support from the knowledge that their loved ones were cared for in their absence. For example, elderly Mrs. Smith was first admitted for radiation therapy following surgery for lung cancer. She went home for a short while, then died during her second admission. Her daughter sent the following note to the staff after the death.

To the staff of EH II

It is extremely difficult for me to adequately put into words the deep gratitude I feel toward the nurses, the aides, and all those in the oncology unit who so lovingly cared for my mother during her last days.

You are, indeed, a special breed, performing not only regular duties but supplying that extra word or touch or presence that meant so very, very much to a suffering and frightened woman. God bless you all and the lives of all you touch.

Very shortly, we will be making a donation to the building fund of the new oncology wing of Charles Medical Center in the hopes that in some small way others might find a degree of comfort and healing.

In loving gratitude,

Gertrude Butler

Mrs. Butler also wrote a newspaper feature article on Father Joe, emphasizing how much his visits brightened her mother's day and noting that they were not of the same religion.

Mr. Cirri, who had inoperable lung cancer, was transferred from another hospital for radiation therapy. He had considerable pain and required oxygen for shortness of breath. Though he never left his bed without a portable oxygen supply, he made it a point to tell almost everyone he spoke with that he had no fears. To the researcher, also, he stressed this, adding that the only fear he had was for his family coming into this section of the city at night. He gave a vivid description of the location of the tumor, which was "too close to the hangar" (the mainstem bronchus) for surgical treatment and explained that he had been all prepared for surgery, when the doctors decided it was too risky.

Mr. Cirri's appearance of bravado was accepted by the staff as his way of coping. One of the Charles nursing students had recognized Mr. Cirri from his visits to a nursing home where she had worked part time as an aide. Mr. Cirri did not disclose to his doctors or the nursing staff that his brother had died in the nursing home from a malignant brain tumor after a slow, traumatic downhill course. After his discharge, Mr. Cirri sent a handwritten letter to Dr. Jones, the chief executive officer, which said, in part:

> . . . I believe Dr. Fisher, the complete medical staff, including your maintenance people, should be highly commended. They made my stay which was a very serious one as pleasant and comfortable as possible. . . . also very helpful is your Radiation Department. . . . This comparison has been made by me from so many stays at different hospitals that were rated as good hospitals that didn't live up to their expectations.

Dr. Jones replied to Mr. Cirri's letter, writing: ". . . I have been at Charles a relatively short time, but it has been long enough to develop a very real respect for our employees and their competence and dedication to qualify medical care. . . ."

After reading the letters, the researcher commented to the head nurse, "Dr. Jones categorizes all care as medical care."

Karen, socialized in a hospital school, indicated that she didn't understand the comment. After further explanation, Karen asked, "You mean you think he should separate nursing care from medical care? Later, Annette, socialized in a baccalaureate program that stressed the autonomy of the nursing profession, commented, "Some of us were pretty upset by that letter."

At one point in Mr. Cirri's hospitalization, the staff thought that if they transferred Mr. Tallini into Mr. Cirri's room, the morale of both men would improve, since both were first-generation Italian-Americans. Mr. Tallini, a seventy-year-old man with multiple myeloma, was recovering from an episode of gastrointestinal bleeding.

After the transfer, no one was able to explain Mr. Tallini's change from being a quiet, anxious person to an aggressively amorous one. The change started one morning when he grabbed and kissed a volunteer, the wife of one of the cardiologists. Despite an understanding but firm approach by the nursing staff, he persisted in grabbing, hugging, and kissing any female who ventured into the three-bed room. At first the staff found his behavior humorous, but as it persisted they found it offensive, since they were intercepted each time they went down the hall. Dr. Fisher's and Father Joe's talks with him only produced apologies and pleas of "Don't tell my wife," but to the nursing staff he insisted, "My wife would understand." The problem was resolved only when Mr. Tallini's family came to take him home, considerably improved.

DECISIONS AND DYING

Death was usually a quiet event preceded by a period of gradually increasing unconsciousness. When a patient died, the bed was curtained off, and after relatives left, post-mortem care was performed. On the day shift, aides or LPN students would occasionally be called to the unit, and the instructor would demonstrate the procedure to the group. Transporters were called to take the body to the morgue. If a patient died around mealtime and the body was still in the room, staff usually served the other patient's meal in the conference room or at the more spacious end of the corridor.

Roommates reacted to the dead or dying in various ways. Mrs. Knull went behind the deceased Mrs. Georgetti's bedside curtain and prayed awhile. A night nurse's note described Valerie Whelan as "inconsolable" after her roommate, Mrs. Raymond, died during the night. The researcher was told that Valerie had expressed annoyance at being awakened frequently during the night by Mrs. Raymond's calls for the nurse. When Valerie realized how sick Mrs. Raymond must have been, she felt terribly guilty about her annoyance. When Mrs. Harris' roommate died, she told the researcher, "Oh, it was a crime; she died during the night and no one was with her."

There were no tabulated data regarding immediate causes of death. In the researcher's opinion, infection, organ failure (hepatic coma, respiratory failure, central nervous system failure), and carcinomatosis (malignancy disseminated to almost all vital organs) were the most common phenomena preceding death in those with slow dying trajectories. In the absence of autopsy data, relatively sudden deaths were thought by the doctors to be caused by embolic phenomena or cardiac arrhythmias; hemorrhage claimed a few patients. But there were exceptions.

Mr. Crosby was an elderly, blind, black man admitted from a county hospital for radiation therapy for lung cancer. He had a few relatives in the area, but none of the staff saw anybody visiting him. Mr. Crosby expectorated large amounts of bronchial secretions into tissues, but because of his blindness, he frequently missed the disposal bag taped to his siderail, and it was common for the soiled tissues to accumulate on the floor. The staff did get Mr. Crosby into a wheelchair and left him in the hall by the nurses' station for a short while each day for some diversion. When the researcher returned to the unit after being away for three days, she was surprised to find that he had died. She asked Annette what he had died from.

"Probably refusal. Two days ago he told Thomas and Long to stop everything. He'd had enough and was ready to die. He refused to eat, drink, or cough. His lungs probably filled up."

The researcher asked, "The doctors went along with his request?"

"Yes," said Annette.

"Was that a surprise?" asked the researcher.

"Yes, it was," responded Annette.

Around noon one day Mr. Jamison suddenly became critically ill, and the head nurse was asked by an LPN to come quickly. Karen checked him, and he looked so bad that she went out to the desk to call the doctor, the man's daughter, and Father Joe. While she was making these calls, the man's roommate called the wife and told her that her husband had died. Karen was surprised and quite embarrassed about the way the wife was notified. Since the body was still in the room, she suggested to the roommate that he eat his lunch in the hall, but he felt quite comfortable about eating in the room.

During the morning report one Sunday, a man came to the nurses' station and said his father, Mr. Breen, needed to be suctioned. Mildred replied that somebody would check him after report. The researcher had gotten to the unit after the report had started but was quite uncomfortable that no one accompanied the son back to the room and checked the father right away. Since she had been away for a few days, she decided to observe rather than intervene. After report, Lisa went down to the man's room, where five relatives were standing around the bed. The patient's oxygen mask wasn't moving. Lisa checked his pulse, then went to the desk and asked Karen to come with a stethoscope. Karen listened for a heartbeat and, hearing none, took off the oxygen mask and looked at the family. They realized Mr. Breen had died.

The curtain had been drawn between the two beds, and the other patient was sleeping. Three of the family members had been there throughout the night, and two had arrived at five in the morning. Lisa took the family to the conference room to wait for the chaplain. Soon she came out of the kitchen with five cups of coffee on a tray.

The head nurse had called for the intern to pronounce Mr. Breen dead, and forty minutes later, she called again. Shortly after that, a sleepy-looking foreign intern in baggy green scrub clothes shuffled onto the unit and asked, "What room?" Karen told him. The researcher waited briefly for Karen to finish what she was doing and then followed her down the hall. Both realized simultaneously that the intern had gone behind the wrong curtain and was standing next to the very cachectic, though fortunately sleeping, roommate. Karen signaled to the intern to go to the other bed. When she got back to the nurses' station, Karen laughingly told Lisa what had almost happened, breaking the tension of the death situation at the start of a long, hard day. It seemed ironic to the researcher that despite the acknowledgments of Mr. Breen's death by his family and the nurses who cared for him, only a total stranger on the bottom rung of the medical hierarchy had the authority to say that he was indeed dead.

The nursing staff consensus was that patients used the words "death" and "dying" infrequently but indicated in other ways that they knew their life was coming to a close. One older woman told a nurse, on her readmission, "I've made my peace with God, but I'm doing this for my family so that they'll be ready and know that they've done all they could."

Marge Holland had a large support system consisting of her mother and seven brothers and sisters as well as close sisters-in-law and brothers-in-law. She did not disclose her feelings about death to the staff, though she told Father Joe that she regretted her mother having to go through this so soon after her father's death five months previously. Several men sobbed as they expressed their sorrow that they would not be able to nurture their children to adulthood.

Vivian, Father Joe, and Janet, the nursing student who had cancer, thought patients would talk about dying and death to anyone who would listen. Vivian said, "I heard a patient talking to the housekeeper saying she didn't want to be a burden. She used to feel that persons who tried to commit suicide were cowards, but now she understands why. She doesn't want to be a burden on her son or her sister."

"Do you think that was a threat?" asked the researcher.

Vivian replied, "I would say she bears watching. She went downstairs before and refused the scans the doctor ordered but got talked into it."

The researcher inquired, "Does anybody besides the housekeeper and yourself know about this?"

"Not so far, but I'll tell Mrs. Foster [Karen] about it," said Vivian.

The aides, Jill and Alice, were both religious persons. Jill thought Alice was the best spiritual adviser on the unit, giving help to families and patients who were not part of a formal religious community. Both were requested by patients to pray with them. Jill thought patients spoke more of an afterlife than of impending death. "I dream of how nice it's going to be," was the way Mr. Christoforo put it.

Mr. Locke, a seventy-nine-year-old patient of Dr. Fisher, had had surgery at Charles for cancer of the colon several years before this admission, and his wife had died of cancer there one year before. Since her death, he had maintained a home and had spent some time in California with a nice. Another niece was a registered nurse at Charles. Mr. Locke was admitted with abdominal metastasis, ascites, and an intestinal obstruction. The doctors conceded that radiation wouldn't help him, but bypass surgery would relieve the pain from the obstruction and make him more comfortable. He was receiving intravenous fluids because oral fluids gave him considerable distress. On rounds one day he said to Dr. Fisher, "Just slowly take away the IV and let me die."

Dr. Fisher said, "I'll do what you want, but I'll let you talk to your family before you make that decision. Your niece is flying in from California." Dr. Fisher wrote on Mr. Locke's chart, "He understands his circumstances and wishes no further treatment. Will await arrival of niece and if then still doesn't want surgery will discontinue IVs."

Mr. Locke agreed to surgery, but his postoperative course was complicated by wound infection and another obstruction. He slowly lost strength and consciousness and died with his nieces at his bedside. They were dressed to go to Mr. Locke's sister's funeral, scheduled for an hour after he died. His nieces said that all of Mr. Locke's business, household, and financial affairs were brought to closure before he had come to the hospital.

The Diehls had a difficult family decision to make. Mr. Diehl, in his sixties, had cancer of the thyroid, and the tumor was compressing his trachea, making it difficult to breathe. It became evident that he would die slowly of asphyxia or require an endotracheal tube and mechanical ventilation. He could not have a tracheostomy because of the location of the tumor. Anticipating an emergency, Dr. Fisher wanted anesthesiologists and equipment readily available. He advised Mr. and Mrs. Diehl, together and separately, and their children also, that Mr. Diehl could live on the respirator, but that eventually they would have to decide when to turn off the machine. Dr. Fisher's office nurse told the researcher that he said to the Diehls, "I'll do what you want, but I want you to make the decision." After some time for consideration, the family decided not to give consent for mechanical breathing. Mr. Diehl received oxygen, sedation, and medication for pain relief and died a quiet death.

Barry Green and his family also had a major decision to make, but Barry was only thirty-five, married, with a five-year-old son. A year before this admission for an intestinal obstruction, Barry had had a malignant tumor removed from his colon, and a colostomy was done. The colostomy was closed three months prior to the new obstruction, but intra-abdominal and liver metastases were noted at surgery. Dr. Fisher ordered a Cantor tube for conservative management of the obstruction, but the tube was not advancing. The surgeons who were called in to examine him wanted to operate; Barry vacillated but finally consented to surgery.

The researcher was on rounds with Dr. Fisher and his office nurse on another unit when Dr. Fisher was paged. The message was that Barry's wife, mother-in-law, and minister were on the Oncology Unit and wanted to speak to Dr. Fisher. On the way to the unit Midge described Barry's wife as obese and "emotional" and stated that the stress of Barry's initial diagnosis and treatment had precipitated a cardiac arrest in the wife, necessitating resuscitation and hospitalization.

On the unit, Barry's wife, with the support of her mother and her minister, told Dr. Fisher that they did not want Barry to undergo more surgery and that this had been decided with Barry before his admission to the hospital. The group went to Barry's bedside. After speaking with them all, Dr. Fisher went to the desk and called the operating room, where the surgeons were waiting. He said to the surgical consultant, "I laid the cards on the table. I told him the surgery would not necessarily prolong his life, but it could make him more comfortable after the immediate postop period. The family knows his prognosis. They want to try to advance the Cantor tube."

Earlier, Dr. Fisher had written on Barry's chart, "Has already had two cycles of the most effective and aggressive program of chemotherapy available with progression of the disease." After the surgery was cancelled, Dr. Fisher wrote that Barry was "fully aware of prognosis but remains hopeful of miracle. Cantor tube not advancing itself but seems to be draining well." Some nurses questioned whether cancelling the surgery was really Barry's decision. He told one staff nurse member, "I only signed the consent for my family."

After the decision to cancel the surgery, Barry withdrew, shunning conversation with anyone and asking only for essentials, such as a urinal or medication for pain or that the Cantor tube be irrigated. He rejected his minister, and even Alice, the aide, a long-time friend and fellow church member. He stopped watching TV, which for awhile had offered him some diversion. At Ted's conference Barry was described as "just laying back there waiting to die. It's eerie because he's so quiet." Occasionally he would make a comment indicating that he had not accepted his condition as terminal. For example, after dreaming that he had a bowel movement, he asked his wife to pray for that. One day he told the head nurse as she was adjusting his IV that he couldn't wait to sink his teeth into something good to eat.

Watching Barry "die by inches," as Dr. Fisher described him, over a two-month period, was difficult for the staff. Even Dr. Fisher looked anguished as he asked daily, "Is there anything that I can do for you?"

Rita, who was new to the unit at the time, questioned why Dr. Fisher just didn't stop the IV; "It's just feeding the tumor," she said. Midge, who made rounds regularly with Dr. Fisher, replied that the IV was Barry's request. He knew he couldn't get along without the Cantor tube without having fecal vomiting, and the IVs were given for hydration only.

Barry's wife, who visited for long periods every day, felt the strain of sitting by his bedside without verbal communication with him, though he was awake. As the weeks went on she made comments about the strain, saying, for example, that when this was all over she wanted to take a long trip. Staff understood this but reacted negatively to some of her behavior, such as eating a hoagie and potato chips at Barry's bedside.

The researcher often observed Barry apparently sleeping with his arms up in the air. He was not aware of her presence unless she touched his hands, and if he awakened he seemed unaware of the posture. Not having an explanation for this phenomenon, she asked several staff members if they could explain it. Only the aide, Alice, could. She said that she thought Barry was praying as they did in their church, according to Psalm 62, verse 5: "Thus I will bless you while I live; lifting up my hands, I will call upon your name."

The week before Barry died, he told his wife he had been praying the wrong way and asked her to pray that the Lord would take him. He asked to see his five-year-old son, and two nights before he died, asked for his minister. A group from his church, including Alice, came and prayed with him and his wife. He told one of the Charles students, "I've found peace within myself, and I'm ready to die."

Two months earlier after the discussion about canceling Barry's surgery, the group had gone across the hall with Dr. Fisher to see Mr. Rinehart, who was deeply jaundiced and semicomatose. He had been transferred from his local hospital to Dr. Fisher's care. Mrs. Rinehart couldn't accept the fact that her husband was dying from cancer of the pancreas and that nothing except comfort measures could be done for him. Dr. Fisher concurred; nothing definitive could be done. A niece from Florida, a registered nurse, was taking care of Mr. Rinehart, whose long-haired, twenty-year-old son, Ricky, was at the bedside. Putting his arm around Ricky's shoulder, Dr. Fisher told him to let the nurses know if his dad became restless or had pain so they could give him something to keep him comfortable. Tears streamed down Ricky's face, and his cousin, the nurse, took hold of him. As the researcher walked away with Dr. Fisher, he commented, somewhat shaken, "It's been an emotional morning."

Two days later when the researcher returned to the unit, Vicki groaned and said:

> It's a good thing you weren't here when Mr. Rinehart died. You would have had something for your study. After he died, his wife and sons made a terrible commotion in the hall outside the nurses' station, crying and wailing. A patient was in the conference room, so we couldn't bring them there. We took them into the utility room. I had to take medication prescribed by Dr. Fisher to all of them.

The new ward clerk, Kate, said, "I think when young boys carry on like that they have something to hide or they're ashamed of something. What do you think?" she asked the researcher, who replied, "Perhaps their cultural background encourages a loud, emotional release at the time of a death."

Vivian said, "I don't agree with you, Kate. I have a friend on South 7 who said those sons were very attentive and stayed with their father the whole time he was there on an earlier admission."

Kate said, "That doesn't mean they didn't feel guilty or something."

Libby added, "You never saw such confusion in all your life. This floor is getting more confusing all the time."

Alice had taken care of a large number of dying patients, but Flo Hamill's death seemed to really upset her. Flo was forty-seven, a very obese woman with lung cancer and metastasis to the spine and bladder. She had bladder spasms and a great deal of pain, and she had no use of her lower extremities. Flo's response to radiation was better than anticipated, with some relief of pain and muscle spasm. One day Dr. Fisher suggested to her that they make plans for her discharge. He said, "It's time to think of a place for your convalescence. You could go home with a visiting nurse to come in daily."

Flo replied, "I need twenty-four-hour care, and I can't pay for nurses."

"You have Major Med?" Dr. Fisher asked.

She answered, "I think so. My husband looked into the Harbor Nursing Home so my twelve-year-old son could walk over and visit."

"I'll talk to Ben about it," said Dr. Fisher. Flo reminded him, "Wherever I go they have to know I go to the bathroom in a Chux pad. They have to have at least LPNs, because I need injections for pain."

"I'll talk to Ben about it," said Dr. Fisher.

Before plans could be completed, however, Flo's pain became worse and she was put on more frequent doses of narcotics. For a month before she died she was described by various members of the staff as "whacked out," "spacey," and "in a drugged state."

One day, Alice came out to the desk from Flo's room about three o'clock, looking very tired. Shortly after she sat down, the team leader came to the desk and said that Flo had died. That surprised Alice and she went back into the room. After that day she made several comments about Flo's death. The researcher asked what she found so troubling about it. Alice said:

> I took care of her for her last three days. Funny, she had less pain and could move better than before, but she couldn't speak—she tried but nothing came out. She complained about the belt tightening around her lower ribs—that's about the sixth patient with spinal involvement who had that complaint. After she died she didn't look peaceful, like most. She actually looked grotesque.

When the researcher returned to the unit following a brief vacation, Mildred Hayes was in charge of the unit and was eager to tell the researcher about the Jasons. Mildred recalled that Jim Jason and his wife Emily had been full of hope and fight until two days before he died. That day Jim hemorrhaged and the staff called Emily in. Mildred recalled that Emily said, "In the past two days we have detected a change in the attitude of the staff and the doctors that you have given up hope."

Mildred replied, "Not given up hope, but we have grave concern for you as part of our family."

Emily sobbed and put her arms around Mildred, saying, "Perhaps the reason God has made my husband so sick is to encounter people like you. I have a great faith in Jesus Christ, and I will never give up hope."

This was Jim Jason's second admission. He was a forty-five-year-old man of imposing stature, weighing 280 pounds. He had been transferred to Dr. Long's care after surgery for cancer of the colon, and on his first admission, in addition to the colostomy, he had multiple, draining abscesses on his abdomen. Though most of the staff had positive regard for Jim, some found him to be abrupt, demanding, and critical. Some accepted this as his way of coping with his illness and did not get too upset by it. Others were affected negatively by his manner. Vivian and Julie couldn't cope with him on his first admission and asked not to be assigned to him. In describing some of the difficulties she had working on EH II, Vivian, a black LPN, said:

> Take that man in 210, Jim Jason. I had him for three days. It just seemed that nothing I did for him was good enough. It got to a point where I didn't like the man.
>
> When he first came, he had these ulcers on his abdomen. They were foul-smelling and looked horrible. I was team leader. The team member would ask me how do you do this. He would say, "Why don't you go ask somebody else who knows what she's talking about." I went to the head nurse; I thought it was a racial thing. Every time I went in he was snappy. I got to feel if nothing I can do for you is any good then I will stay away from you. Even the temporary clerk—he really snapped at her. She's black, too. She asked him his name to give him his mail. The head nurse said, "Maybe you're right." Racism has never popped up before, but it really got to me. I know this. I can feel it. I'm from the South.

"You've felt this before?" asked the researcher.

> Yes, but it's never been so overt. He has his own way of doing things. He's demanding. We were doing it the way it should have been done. The way the doctor wanted it. We finally did what he wanted, but also the way it should have been done.
>
> But that other thing—I knew what it was.

Mildred, the charge nurse, told the staff at the desk one day that Jim was being readmitted "to be put on the intrahepatic pump for chemotherapy."

"That's the end of him," said June.

"It doesn't do anybody any good," Libby added.

The plan was to take Jim to surgery to close his colostomy and insert the arterial catheter. The day before surgery, the researcher was talking to Jim when Dr. Long came in. Talking about his colostomy to Dr. Long, Jim said, "I want to get it out. It's been there since Easter."

Dr. Long replied, "That's already been decided. Don't go back over your tracks." Jim was being prepared for the surgery with colostomy irrigations, enemas, and blood transfusions. He was supposed to have nothing by mouth, but asked Dr. Long if he could have a bowl of his wife's homemade potato soup. He also asked Dr. Long to bring in the specifications for his sports car so he could determine what was causing the car's problem. This would give him something to keep his mind occupied the morning of surgery. Dr. Long said he would, but didn't. After the doctor left, Jim commented, with tears in his eyes, "This is some society. They're all such good people. They are great."

Emily took her husband the potato soup, which she had warmed in the kitchen. Their relationship was admired by the staff; as one member commented, "The husband and wife discussed everything openly until he became semicomatose the day before his death. No matter how gross his body looked, neither ever indicated the slightest negativity about it."

Jim's surgeon came to the nurses' station the day after surgery to tell the staff that Jim was doing better. The hepatic catheter had not been inserted at surgery because he had hemorrhaged. The surgeon formed his hands into a huge scoop and gestured as he described three basins full of cancerous material that was removed from Jim's abdomen. He had some liver metastasis but not as much as expected. The colostomy was closed. Because his condition required close monitoring, Jim was transferred to the Intensive Care Unit, where he stayed for about two weeks. His condition warranted his remaining there, but he pleaded with the doctors to send him back to EH II. He complained about the staff attitudes in the ICU, particularly on the night shift.

The supervisor, Frances, said, "You know how the nurses horse around to relieve some of the tension. He thought that was very unprofessional. He even referred to one member of the nursing staff as an addict."

"Well, I made it back," a thinner and jaundiced Jim said as his stretcher passed the nurses' station.

Despite their concern for the Jasons, the EH II staff was upset by the added work. The number and timing of observations and the care involved with the tubes, catheters, pumps, drainage vessels, IVs, transfusions, and dressings necessitated that one staff member be assigned solely to Jim. In addition, because of his size and all the appendages, three people were sometimes required to turn him.

It was close to Christmas, and holiday time off further depleted the work force; no replacements had been made for the two experienced RNs who had left. Staff griped to the supervisor that other patients were getting less attention and would be complaining. For example, Mr. Richards, an elderly man with lung cancer, who had been admitted for the third time in several months, was in the bed near Jim Jason's in the three-bed room. When a staff member was with Mr. Richards, his mind was quite clear. However, he would talk to himself when nobody was giving him direct attention. This bothered Jim, and he asked the staff to keep Mr. Richards occupied, but one of the major reasons they couldn't do that was because they were so busy with Jim.

The Jasons had three children, the oldest a sixteen-year-old daughter. When his condition was worsening, Jim told June, the registered nurse who was assigned to him, that he would like to hold his daughter. But with all the tubes and drainage, the girl was afraid to come near him. June spread a clean sheet across his chest so that he could hold his daughter without her coming into contact with the profuse drainage. June observed that the daughter seemed uncomfortable with this show of affection.

Jim died about five weeks after surgery. His wife, mother, and daughter were with him and left the unit about midnight. Mildred concluded her description of what she regarded as the "most difficult patient situation the unit ever had," by saying:

> Dr. Long was unreal. Jim was in a coma for the last twelve hours, and Long wouldn't let us turn off the IVs. That clears the infection, you know.

> As Jim got progressively worse, the surgeon wanted to feed him by hyper-alimentation. I told him, "Dr. Pauson, you wouldn't dare." His partner, a female surgeon, told me not to let Dr. Pauson go back there to Jim's room. Dr. Pauson was so guilt-ridden that he stood by Jim and gave him sips of water. Food was coming through the midline incision. Two days before he died, Jim bled heavily through the midline incision. Ice chips even came through it. Ruth, who was assigned to Jim that day, couldn't cope with the "big bleed." The day before he died Dr. Long pointed out that Jim's bilirubin was at an improved level. Right up to the last he would not acknowledge that Jim was getting worse.

A short while later Dr. Long brought in a lengthy letter from Emily Jason expressing her gratitude to him for all he did for Jim and stating her belief that Jim had died with grace and dignity. She returned to the unit a month after Jim's death with some cookies and a thank-you letter for the nursing staff on the three shifts. She told the head nurse that while the family was at Jim's funeral, their house had been broken into and robbed of money and valuables.

Jim Jason was not the only patient who had a difficult time in the Intensive Care Unit. Rachel Brown, an attractive fifty-two-year-old blonde, had cancer of the gall bladder, which was removed eighteen months prior to her admission for radiation therapy for marked liver metastasis. Rachel explained that after she went home following the radiation therapy she felt fairly good and did not want to take the oral narcotic for pain that Dr. Fisher had prescribed. She thought it was too strong, so she started taking aspirin when she had pain. "I should have known better because I had an ulcer and bleeding a few years ago," she said. "I just never thought of the aspirin starting the bleeding now."

Rachel was pale and receiving transfusions, but as always, she looked chic and well groomed. "You always wonder," she said, "is this it?" Rachel had been admitted to another unit at Charles, and though she had some complaints about EH II on her first admission, she begged Dr. Fisher to transfer her to EH II. She described the care on the other unit as "horrendous."

Studies failed to disclose the point of Rachel's bleeding. She was treated with transfusions when her daily hemoglobin and hematocrit reports were low. One morning she felt well enough to get to the bathroom for a shower. While there, she became weak and vomited blood. Late that night she had a severe transfusion reaction. Since she required close observation around the clock, Rachel was transferred to Intensive Care. Dr. Fisher wrote on the chart, "This lady is a CODE candidate," but he had to hold a conference with the ICU staff, who could not understand the rationale for treating a patient with cancer and liver metastasis in Intensive Care.

A few days later the researcher went to visit Rachel in the ICU, a huge rectangular room with a rectangular nurses' station in the center. Only cloth curtains were used when necessary to separate one bed from the next, so patients could readily observe much of what was happening to others. Rachel was receiving a variety of therapies in an attempt to stop the bleeding. As Dr. Fisher phrased it, "We have pulled out all the magic potions in the bag of tricks." But she continued to bleed. She was awaiting the arrival of donor-related platelets from her son and her brother in California. She was still her witty, observant self, but she was upset by the care she received on the night shift. She said:

> There is a color line here. The three black aides on the night shift wouldn't offer to help me, but they help the black girl in the next bed without even being asked. With my both hands tied down with the blood and IV, they wouldn't even offer to clean me after I got off the bedpan. I couldn't even help myself. I complained about them one night because they were so noisy. So they stopped talking, but they rolled their chairs the rest of the night— they know the chairs have this squeaky noise when you roll them. I have a saying for them . . . "See no pain, hear no pain, feel no pain."

The researcher mentioned this incident to Karen, who had worked nights in the Intensive Care Unit. Karen remarked that the same thing was going on then, but that the supervisor didn't do any thing about it.

Rachel Brown did not respond to the donor-related platelets. She was transferred to a major medical center for surgery to induce clotting in her gastrointestinal tract but died there shortly after the operation. The word got back to Charles that the bleeding had resulted from radiation reaction in the internal tissues, but the nursing staff remarked that the Charles radiologist had said this was "impossible."

Generally, nurses were impressed that so many patients put up such a tremendous fight for life. As Lisa noted, "Mr. Reardon, I thought for sure he was going to die two months before he did—and I'm sure there was something in him that he didn't want to die."

Jill, a newcomer to the health-care field, observed, "Some grasp on to what life they have and adapt so well. You come to admire yourself as a human species that can grow and adapt to all kinds of adverse situations." The captain expressed continual amazement that the greatest concern of so many patients was the heartbreak and strain their illness brought to others.

In a tribute to a woman who died of cancer after a ten-year, day-by-day struggle with all the afflictions of the disease and its treatment, a newspaper columnist observed that the price of survival—pain, discomfort, indignity, helplessness, disfigurement, and fear—"seem more than a person would reasonably want to bear." But he went on to state that in "our narrow notion of life" we shrink from illness and unpleasantness and eye such realities as cancer with a medieval dread. We look at cancer patients and wonder why they don't give up. And the lesson that he learned from a courageous woman was that, "All life is terminal. Yet it is fully ours until the last of it is gone. Only then is there death. Not a moment before" [1].

REFERENCES

1. Kilian, M. Aunt Jule, a story of courage. *Philadelphia Inquirer,* 6 November 1977, p. 5-F.

Chapter 7
Summary, Conclusions, and Recommendations

SUMMARY

This ethnographic research has provided an opportunity to examine typical problems, norms of behavior, manifest role patterns, and the structure of social relations and interactional patterns on an oncology unit in a community general hospital. Particular attention has been given to the role behavior of registered nurses; the coping mechanisms employed by nurses in this subculture; and personal, social, and institutional variables that contribute to the perpetuation of nurses' current behavior patterns. Raw data have been extensively used because of the clarity with which members of the subculture stated their view of their situation.

Since nurses are the largest group of health care providers in American society, their education can be viewed as a significant factor in the quality of health care. This study also provided an opportunity to examine some aspects of the basic and continuing education of registered nurses, the American system of health care delivery, and nurses' roles in maintaining hospital subsystems. Institutional constraints are identified that inhibit nurses from providing the best quality nursing care to cancer patients and their families. The significance of education as a route to lessening those constraints is addressed also. Attention has been given to patients and families, the doctors, hospital administration, structural and functional aspects of the hospital, the Oncology Unit, and related hospital departments.

CONCLUSIONS

Overall, in the view of the researcher, patients admitted to the Oncology Unit at Charles Hospital were in a humane and caring environment. This was certainly true by comparison with the rest of the hospital, according to patients, doctors, and nurses from different units. Doctors came and went, spending only a brief period daily with each patient. Hospital administrators communicated only through their memos. On the other hand, individual registered nurses, and the nursing staff under their direction, spent a minimum of eight hours a day providing care for patients in an environment that many members of American society would find frightening. Members of the nursing service were the only group providing care for patients twenty-four hours a day, seven days a week. Their low-salaried work involved tasks that many people would regard as distressing, demeaning, distasteful, or even disgusting, and physically exhausting as well. Care was provided within the "situation-limits" conditions of individual patients' grief, solitude, anxiety, anger, depression, suffering, dying, and death.

The serious nursing responsibilities related to sickness, treatment, suffering, death, and patient and family crises were assumed by women of diverse educational and experiential backgrounds, whose ages ranged from the early twenties to the late sixties. The staff usually functioned at a fast pace, fully occupied with their immediate tasks. Urgent physical care requirements often took precedence over other important aspects of care, such as listening to patients. There was neither time nor space for reflective thinking or long-range planning.

The work of the nursing staff on an oncology unit is highly demanding in both instrumental and expressive aspects. Registered nurses were best prepared for and most skilled at the instrumental aspects of care, and these aspects were also what the system expected of them and held them accountable for. They tended to ignore or avoid other aspects of care in which they lacked both theoretical preparation and skill, such as systematic assessment and writing plans for nursing care.

Nursing staff at Charles most often acted on the premise that talking, listening, teaching, and providing diversion to patients were activities to be done only if there was time after baths, medications, and treatments. The realities of the staffing pattern sometimes made it necessary for them to set these priorities in their work. Some staff members expressed guilt feelings about having yielded time for talking to other exigencies, only to find that for the patient, there was no further opportunity. With cancer patients, particularly, nurses should not have to put off exploring the emotional components of their stage of illness. In fact, opportunities for interaction should be deliberately furnished, if care of cancer patients is to be consonant with the institution's and the Department of Nursing's pronouncements about the goals of patient care.

The anger of patients and family members at each other, and the anger of patients and doctors at the nursing staff, posed particular difficulties. Yet registered nurses did not seek out specific help to deal with their own anger or that of patients, families, and doctors.

Other recurrent themes were doctors' denials and their intraprofessional conflicts, as well as the conflict generated by bioethical dilemmas, such as the nursing staff's perception of the overaggressive treatment of patients close to death. Added to the other anxiety-producing factors in this setting, such conflict situations naturally reduced the staff's capacity to be inventive or versatile in resolving patient care problems. While day staff derived some assistance from the support conferences with the head nurse from the Psychiatric Unit, these were perceived by some staff members as too unfocused and infrequent for the kind of help they needed. Nevertheless, staff did not clamor for additional help. Basically, they accepted the situation as given.

Work Stresses

Patient care in the hospital was organized on a part-task, bureaucratic system. Speed, efficiency, cooperation, loyalty to the institution, and adherence to externally imposed rules and regulations were highly valued, although supplies and other means necessary to achieve certain goals were sometimes lacking, due to deficiencies in other hospital departments.

Organizational, professional-bureaucratic, and interpersonal conflicts generated a great deal of tension and job dissatisfaction. The turnover of registered nurse staff, uninspired recruitment techniques, lack of replacements for nurses who resigned, and the eventual employment of part-time nurses to replace full-time staff resulted in instability within the supposed leadership group of registered nurses on the Oncologic Unit. The values of the hospital administration interfered in other ways, also; because a ward clerk was not hired for several months, the head nurse or charge nurse had to spend her time on clerical work rather than on nursing management, supervision, and development of nursing staff. Additional stress was caused by organizational restructuring, including the introduction and eventual withdrawal (demanded by physicians) of a more patient-oriented record system.

Interdepartmental boundary disputes that affected the Oncology Unit often had to be resolved by the nursing supervisor and the head nurse. The supervisor also had to compensate for the deficiencies of other departments, as by checking that lids were on garbage cans and that doctors signed their orders, or by delivering administrative memos. Although the head nurse and supervisor complained about these non-nursing tasks, they did so only to other nurses, thus demonstrating that they were willing to go along with the system. Nurses did not exhibit an individual or collective professional self-concept consonant with the importance of their contribution to patient care or hospital system maintenance. Additionally, it was as if the first glimmer of the women's liberation movement had yet to reach Charles Hospital.

Hours of Work

Family and social activities in American society are timed around the usual working day. For this reason, hospital work on the evening and night shifts has less status than work during the day. At the same time, work on these shifts is often more difficult, because there are fewer staff and the work is unrelieved by variety.

At Charles, not only were the hours inconvenient, but travel within the inner city and weather conditions were perceived as dangerous and sometimes hazardous. Another deficiency of working these shifts was the lack of educational opportunities, which, though few, were generally planned for the day shift. Although there was a small salary differential for work on these shifts, greater incentives would make such working hours more attractive, so that units could be more regularly staffed, particularly during the night shift. Innovative approaches might include having one position shared by two cooperating nurses or providing for a four-night work week with full employee benefits, instead of the usual five-night week.

Collective Bargaining

Nurses have the legal right to organize and bargain collectively, and state nurses' associations that are affiliates of the American Nurses' Association have the legal authority to act as the bargaining representative for local units. However, head nurses, who are in managerial positions, are caught in a double bind. The head nurse and the supervisor of the Oncology Unit at Charles would be supportive if staff made demands of the administration on practice issues, such as adequate staffing, inservice education, and greater control over decisions affecting nursing care. Yet as part of the hospital management team, the head nurse and supervisor would be on the opposite side of the bargaining table from their staff nursing colleagues. The hospital administration thus limited the autonomy and power of nursing even more, in effect pitting nurse against nurse by "promoting" head nurses to management-titled positions.

The directors of nursing and of inservice education were also in management positions. While they had the authority to speak for nursing and had much to do with the quality of nursing care in the institution, they squelched efforts to promote the ANA at Charles because of its economic and general welfare (bargaining) component. Though nursing staff on the unit verbalized many discontents about the work situation to each other, there was no evidence that they were aware of their right to organize and bargain collectively. None belonged to the professional association. Moreover, staff nurses at Charles Hospital did not have the opportunity to meet collectively during working hours. The directors of nursing and inservice education separately verbalized their repudiation of large group meetings of the nursing staff for educational or other purposes. Although the nurses could have met on their own outside the work environment, this option was not exercised, nor was such a suggestion heard by the researcher.

The Work System of Nurses

Whether or not a nurse had chosen oncology nursing and was commited to it was an important consideration in her work performance and job satisfaction. Some staff members had negative views of cancer, its potential for treatment, and the grouping of cancer patients on one unit. The effect of their attitudes on individual patients was not assessed, but staff members who expressed negative attitudes had a low level of job satisfaction.

Conflicts among the nursing staff members resulted from uneven workloads, differences of opinion between younger and older nurses about nursing practice and education, differences in job preparation and commitment, and differences in opinion about the value of written care plans for patients. Role tension between nurses' aides and RNs and LPNs occurred over issues of patient privacy, unfair workload, unclear role responsibilities of students from various programs, promptness in providing pain medication for patients, and written directives for giving care.

Despite the inherent stresses and tensions, there was group solidarity and a general attitude of openness, cooperation, and commitment to patients among the nursing staff. This attitude contributed to the good spirit and stability of the unit, which in turn contributed to stability in the hospital system. Humor, laughter, sarcasm, cooperation, and group support were identified as the group's major coping mechanisms.

Although registered nurses were relatively powerless with respect to persons of higher status (doctors, administrators), they did not abuse their power over staff persons of lesser status. There seemed to be more manifest discord and disagreement among the registered nurses than among the licensed practical nurses or aides. The relationship of registered nurses to lower-echelon nursing staff, staff from other departments, visitors, and families were for the most part warm and respectful.

The staff were flexible about rules concerning visiting hours, time limits on patients' diversionary activities, lights-out or wake-up hours, and the timing of care activities such as bathing or bedmaking. They did not routinely awaken patients in the early morning hours for such activities as temperature taking. There was evidence that some staff members who were having difficulty coping with job and personal stress acted impatiently with patients. Occasionally, derogatory remarks were made between doctors and nurses or within a nursing staff group about a patient's behavior, with no attempt to understand the behavior or explore its meaning. Patients' complaints about the performance of individual staff members on the same or another shift seemed to be ignored or passed over lightly.

Behaviors that patients might find depersonalizing or dehumanizing were often thoughtless violations of the rules of common courtesy. One kind of depersonalizing behavior was shown when physicians and nurses on rounds discussed treatment plans or held nonprofessional conversations in the presence of patients while excluding their participation. The researcher believed that this was not intentional, but it indicated that the doctor, not the patient or the nurse, was the power person in the nurse-doctor-patient triad.

At all levels some members of the nursing staff were intuitively more sensitive than others. These caring persons, as well as other support persons associated with the unit, were able to provide some support for patients when others could not or did not.

Nursing staff members were in positions of power over patients, particularly with regard to the administration of medication for pain. The problem of providing for pain relief was recurrent, particularly on the night shift, for several reasons, including transiency of night shift and unclear medical orders. However, no effective effort was made to resolve the problem, as by inservice education programs on the management of pain. Some families exerted control over administration of medications by telephoning the doctor directly with complaints about a relative's care.

The three shifts were identified as separate though related subcultures that lacked coordination.

Role Strain

In addition to the inherent stresses associated with the physical, psychologic, and sociocultural aspects of caring for patients with cancer at various stages, other factors contributed to nurses' role strain. The qualities of gentleness, nurturing, and caring that are so necessary for nursing cancer patients led nurses to meet expectations that they meet the needs of other departments and of the doctors as well, often at the cost of time and energy that could be devoted to improving their nursing practice.

The system of power politics in the hospital was intimately intertwined with the work situation on the Oncology Unit. Although the top managerial triad in the Charles Hospital organization included administration, medicine and nursing, nurses were clearly subordinate to both other groups.

Ashley, Grissum and Spengler, Sills, and others point out that several factors account for the relative powerlessness of nurses in the subsystem of the American hospital [1-3]. The position of nurses is highly related to attitudes of men toward women in the work setting and to the primary and secondary socialization of female nurses. First, nursing is almost exclusively a women's profession, and the primary socialization of women in American society has been as passive, conforming, dependent persons, trained for a lifetime as appendages to men. Gentle, nurturing, sensitive behavior is supposedly a natural characteristic of women; a female child who is assertive, logical, analytical, curious, and independent is considered by many to be unnatural and unfeminine [4].

In addition to this primary socialization, the secondary socialization of women in hospital schools of nursing reinforces the traditional, passive feminine role. Ashley asserts that nurses in hospital schools were trained as apprentices, not as professionals [5]. Nurturing qualities and deference to physicians and hospital administrators were highly valued, as were cooperation, faith in those in high-status positions, and self-sacrifice [6]. Intellectual curiosity, innovativeness, and questioning the status quo were considered deviant behaviors.

At Charles Hospital, a general climate of intellectual stagnation in the nursing division and lack of a strong professional identity meant that nurses were subject to the will and whimsies of others, instead of having influence consistent with their degree of responsibility. Lack of a "critical mass" of more autonomously socialized nurses to offset the diploma-school tradition of dependence was an additional deficit.

The intensive enculturation in the hospital training school mentality was demonstrated in this study by nurses' tendencies to be agreeable, self-sacrificing, and nonassertive for the good of the doctors and the hospital. The price they paid for exhibiting these qualities was large: they did not grow in their own professional sphere of influence; they did not adequately supervise lesser-trained nursing workers; they did not pay enough attention to systematic planning and evaluation of nursing care or to coordination throughout the three shifts; there was very limited staff education; and supportive family conferences were discontinued. For the most part, nurses were passive in their relationships with physicians and administrators, accepting what was delegated to them by these two groups, which have traditionally assigned minor roles to nurses. They resented being used in this manner, but they lacked the self-confidence, assertiveness, and other interpersonal skills required to confront persons about issues. They also lacked the time, emotional energy, and the group organizational effort necessary for such tactics. When nurses did recognize that something delegated to them was beyond their scope of responsibility, they ignored the request rather than state their position.

Nurses' Professional Role

Because hospital nursing schools are oriented to a medical model of patient care, nurses from these programs have been trained to implement the orders of physicians. Nurses did not develop skills in problem solving or critical thinking about nursing care problems and issues, and the system did not value these skills as a necessary component of professional nursing behavior. Additionally, nurses in traditional schools were given an occupational or vocational, rather than a professional, view of nursing. Unlike members of other professions, many nurses had minimal interest in nursing as a lifelong field of service or inquiry [7]. They expected to meet society's expectations that women become wives and homemakers.

Except for the new graduates, the registered nurses on Charles' Oncology Unit, as well as members of its supervisory staff and Inservice Education Department, had dropped out of nursing for a significant length of time during the knowledge explosion of the fifties and sixties. Most who returned to nursing did so for economic reasons. Meanwhile, the traditions of Charles Hospital, with its older graduates from the still-operating hospital school, its older doctors, its stringent financial heritage, and its weak staff development structure permitted these nurses to return as if little cognitive change in nursing had occurred in the decade or more of their absence. Role models, in the form of head nurses and supervisors, were unchanged from models of one to four decades previously; staff nurses returning after a long hiatus easily fell into step.

Ideology-Reality Conflict

To the observer, there was considerable disparity between the nursing profession's ideologic pronouncements about the current practice of nursing and the actual role performance of registered nurses at Charles. However, the registered nurses did not seem to experience conflict concerning the profession's statements of their ideal role. Most were unfamiliar with such pronouncements since they were not members of the professional association and had been inactive in nursing during the most active period of the profession's growth. When there was an awareness of conflict between ideology and reality, nurses acted to reduce or eliminate the conflict in several ways. One way was by establishing priorities; a major priorty was the immediate and real goal of accomplishing a certain quantity of work within a certain time and space and within the expectations of people other than the professional nursing subculture.

Other factors interfered with stated or implied nursing goals. The locus of power was in the medical staff, but authority in the form of dicta that nurses were expected to enforce came through the administrative structure. Nurses on the Oncology Unit were sometimes caught between the two groups. These system constraints on nurses, as well as other factors, resulted in lack of freedom to make choices directly affecting their own practice.

Generally, nurses did what they knew how to do best. Rather than undertake areas of responsibility in which they were insecure, such as writing nursing care plans or conducting patient care conferences, they tended to maintain the status quo. Each staff member performed her daily assignment as she thought it should be done, primarily providing basic hygienic and comfort care to patients and carrying out doctors' orders for medication and treatment. Rather than nursing patients toward specific goals, the nurses tended to approach each patient's care in much the same way. Nursing practice seemed largely intuitive rather than based on current theory, as professional ideology advocates. A recent graduate of a baccalaureate nursing program provided a notable, though inconsistent, exception, and occasionally other staff members did also. There was a lack of system in the approach to and evaluation of common problems, such as pain, nutrition, and bowel hygiene. There was little joint planning or evaluation of nursing care, though a nursing audit system was in its initial phase.

Feedback from patients, families, and doctors indicated a degree of satisfaction with this level of care in many cases. However, there was also some feedback that some patients' nursing needs were not being met. Patients with complex physiologic and psychologic needs constituted the difficult group. At times staff expressed dissatisfaction with the level of care they provided, but for the most part, the nurses did not have the theoretical foundation or the access to nursing consultants required to provide more sophisticated care.

Role blurring, or the overlapping of the traditional registered nurses' functions with those of licensed practical nurses and aides, did not cause undue concern among the registered nurses. The aides on the day shift, in the researcher's view, functioned above the general expectations stated in the hospital's job description for workers at this level. The expectations of licensed practical nurses were clearly above their level of formal preparation, particularly with regard to the team leadership role, a function not listed in the job description. Registered nurses generally performed below the level of expectations stated in the hospital's nursing manual and in the nursing profession's standards of practice, with regard to systematic effort to assess, plan (and write the plan), carry out, and evaluate individualized patient care.

Today, the nursing profession's statements of ideal role reflect the view that directors of nursing, nursing supervisors, and head nurses are first and foremost nurses, but also persons who are knowledgeable about management. Their role functions are viewed as primarily concerned with developing and achieving nursing care goals as an integral part of patient care. Hospital administration at Charles acted on the view that the head nurses and nursing supervisors were primarily managers and coordinators of hospital services who were also knowledgeable about the practice of nursing. Doctors, to a large extent, related to nurses as their assistants in delivering medical care rather than as co-professionals with a different area of expertise. With rare exception, nurses at Charles functioned in consonance with the views of administrators and physicians. At times nurses questioned among themselves some of the social implications of the system, but generally felt a lack of resources and power to change it. Especially after the departure of two full-time RNs without replacements, the daily stresses of the work environment made it necessary for the head nurse to go along with the system to keep role strain at a bearable level. She directed her energies to coordinating care that was essential to keep the complaints of doctors, patients, families, and other departments to a minimum and to maintain some stability in the system.

The head nurse had a very demanding position in a complex social system with a multiplicity of interactions and interpersonal relationships. Her decisions had an immediate effect on the life and well-being of patients. It is difficult to envision a hospital administrator with a comparable level of responsibility who would do his secretary's work for four months or mop floor spills because the Housekeeping Department had already done its once-over for the day. Similarly, physicians who are full-time hospital employees do not feel it necessary to do others' work besides their own. A major difference between medical and hospital administrative professionals and the nurses was the nurses' lack of self-identity as co-professionals with rights and responsibilities to make demands, to say "no," or to have autonomy regarding the scope of responsibility of nursing practice, as well as accountability for the knowledge base of nursing practice. But the secondary socialization of the nurse in hospital schools taught her that it was noble to pick up the slack for all other hospital departments as well as for doctors, particularly between sundown and sunrise. Nurses from hospital schools who were in managerial and faculty positions in Charles Hospital and its school of nursing cooperated in perpetuating these values. Meanwhile, the new hospital administrator, concerned primarily with a medical school enterprise supported with a massive infusion of public funds, viewed the continuation of nurse training in the hospital school as a "convenience" for the hospital system. The inadequacies of this mode of education for the individuals it trained and its detrimental effects on patient care were apparently not a consideration.

A nursing supervisor at Charles recognized the need for change in the system but looked to the future group of young, more assertive nurses to make the changes. In addition to being socialized to passivity, a realistic reason for nurses not to press for change was the economic one; all but one of the staff worked out of economic necessity. Nurses who had to work for a living were unwilling to risk losing a job by openly challenging the status quo. Often the supervisor's and head nurse's conflicts between hospital managerial functions and professional nursing functions were resolved in favor of systems maintenance. Some notable exceptions were the supervisor's patient advocacy role in changing the assignment of research-drug monitoring costs from the patient to the pharmaceutical company, and the nurses' recommendation of standing medical orders that they could implement according to their judgment of patients' needs. Nurses were also more flexible in regard to visitor regulations and controlled admissions and transfers within the unit. They also graciously welcomed a nurse researcher into their midst.

Education

In other professions, it is usual to study one's own field in greater depth to prepare for the assumption of greater responsibilities. But because of the stated hardships of travel, time, and money, and probably because of some undervaluation of advanced education in nursing, many graduates of hospital schools who have wanted positions of leadership have obtained baccalaureate degrees in nonnursing majors. When nurses study for credentials in nonnursing majors, the knowledge base of their own professional practice does not expand, and in fact, becomes relatively more constricted. They lack knowledge of advancements in the profession which they would acquire through the study of nursing, and they also lose the opportunity for resocialization through association with professional peers.

In the nursing structure at Charles, the director of inservice education held high status in the system, legitimizing her influence. She had power to be a change agent, but she appeared threatened by her lack of knowledge and the attitudinal gap with younger nurses, because she had left the practice of nursing for some time and had pursued degrees in other fields. As observed by a number of staff persons and by the researcher, her efforts were directed toward the promulgation of inservice programs that emphasized psychomotor skills, such as the dispensing of drugs, but not the requisite theory, related to cancer chemotherapeutic agents or the management of pain, on which to base sound nursing assessment and intervention. She denigrated the state's professional nursing association to her staff and viewed standards of nursing practice as the impositions of accrediting agencies. This devaluation was transmitted downward to nurses at the staff level.

Though the policy manual of Charles mandated nursing care planning and patient care conferences, the lack of any systematic direction and help for the staff in doing this and lack of accountability for these activities revealed how little they were actually valued. Another stress added to those inherent in the work situation for the nurses was the expected change of their role functions to meet accreditation criteria for nursing care planning and evaluation, without the administration providing the requisite time, direction, and assistance to make this change. The high turnover of nurses with new ideas and enthusiasm for nursing in the Inservice Education Department was an indicator of the ineffectiveness of its leadership.

Personal variables. All members of the nursing staff had changing family concerns. During the research year, several of them experienced personal and family crises of serious illness, permanent disability, or death. Because of these crises, they did not seek changes in the work arena, but rather, hoped for some sense of stability in an inherently unstable work situation. They directed their energy to getting through each day. Given the fast work pace and the frequent shortage of staff, there was little time for future planning, and little reward was envisioned for changing the status quo.

Three of the nurses reduced the combined stresses of work and family responsibilities by partial withdrawal through a change from full-time to part-time work, despite the loss of economic rewards. Excessive role strain was manifest in nursing staff at all levels by fatigue, psychosomatic disorders, disturbed interpersonal relationships, and in one case, deviant social behavior on the ward.

Group coping mechanisms and the psychological support derived from the staff conferences with the head nurse from the Psychiatric Unit did seem to have some positive effect. Additionally, members of the staff whose orientation was religious—the two aides and the head nurse—derived support from their beliefs and seemed to obtain greater job satisfaction and to be more able to cope with the stresses. The personal experience of successfully coping with significant loss was identified by several of the staff as a major factor in successful adaptation to working with cancer patients.

Doctors

Although there was more informality and more professional collaboration in the nurse-doctor relationship on this unit than is traditionally the case in hospitals, nurses experienced considerable conflict and feelings of powerlessness in their relationships with physicians. Some problems were related to disagreements about the medical management of the terminally ill; others were related to the absolute autonomy of physicians. Another issue was the injustice of doctors blaming or scolding individual nurses for circumstances beyond their control. But when conflicts arose between the bureaucratic system and physician entrepreneurs, nurses were most tactful in taking the roles of mediator and coordinator between the two subsystems.

One factor adding to the problem of work organization on the unit was the need of doctors to maintain and rebuild their practices. Doctors came to the hospital for rounds and ensuing order changes at times that were convenient to their office schedules, consultation trips, research, and other endeavors; their schedules, at times, did not coincide with the convenience of patients or nurses. Nurses spent quite a bit of time contacting doctors after they left the hospital to clarify orders, get new orders, or report emergent conditions, which contributed to the difficulty of work organization on the unit.

The interpersonal conflicts and lack of communication among the three major admitting physicians also contributed to registered nurse role strain, particularly at the charge nurse level. Registered nurses were very caught up in the physicians' disputes; in the professional conflict between two of the physicians, they functioned as listeners and cheerleaders for the doctor whom they identified as the underdog. They acted as message carriers and interpreters of institutional rules and policies for the physicians, who did not overtly engage in social or professional dialogue with each other.

Only when there was a collective threat to physician autonomy (opposition to integrated progress notes) did the doctors agree on an issue, though their views were expressed individually rather than collectively. The nursing staff highly respected the medical director of the unit as an oncologist, but they resented his failure to deal directly with problems related to medical practice on the unit. His hands-off policy protected the professional autonomy of the physicians but left nurses with no effective recourse. However, at the request of the nurses he did intercede with the nursing administration with regard to staffing and overtime pay, obtained an educational scholarship for the head nurse, offered his office for a learning experience, and arranged to have the unit painted. Still, it was far from being a co-professional model of doctor-nurse relationship, and the value of not interfering with the doctor in his work overrode certain ideals about nurse-patient behavior. The nurses' deference to doctors was illustrated by their failure to volunteer significant nursing information about patients while on rounds, making these medically focused rather than interdisciplinary. A doctor's displeasure or the threat of it created tension that was disruptive of nursing staff morale. When displeasure was evident, the nurses and doctors avoided spontaneous interaction and dialogue, which decreased the sharing of information about patients' needs or problems. Nurses also deferred to doctors by not doing or saying more than was essential in order not to further inflame a situation. Nurses became adept at reading doctors' moods and acting on those readings.

Although nurses' errors were recorded and filed in incident reports, there was no such mechanism for incorrect or inconsistent doctors' orders; nurses intercepted these. Nurses resented being corrected in front of patients for situations the nurses were not involved in and being questioned on obscure medical facts in front of patients. Inhibited from releasing their aggressive feelings directly, nurses dispelled them by joking, sarcasm, or complaining among themselves rather than effecting a confrontation with doctors either in front of patients or alone.

Some of the nursing staff had strong opinions about the approach to treatment of one of the oncologists. They questioned whether certain diagnostic tests or certain treatments that he ordered were useful for a given stage of illness, and whether patients and families were given enough information about certain research drugs and other aspects of treatment. Nurses were directly involved in administering investigational drugs and preparing patients for diagnostic tests and treatments, all of which were orderd by physicians. However, except for occasional weak and timid questioning of the physician, they raised ethical issues only among themselves. The nursing supervisor did confront an issue of unfair costs and successfully resolved this in favor of the patients.

Patients

Despite the hospital's statements that individualized patient care was the goal of the institution, patients were usually passive recipients rather than active participants in their program of care. The capriciousness of the disease of cancer and the vagaries of individual response to treatment made powerlessness a fact of life. Patients' place in the system reinforced this. With their own lives in jeopardy, they felt most safe in going along with the system. Thus, they ignored disagreements between two of the attending physicians, even when the disagreements were overt. Nurses in this situation did not act as patient advocates, but caught in the same medical power struggle, allied themselves with the employed physician who was in disagreement with his employer.

Interdisciplinary dialogue, which should include the patient, was characteristically lacking in the subculture. Frequently only the charge nurse or other registered nurses made rounds with the doctors or talked to the representatives of other departments such as Social Service, Physical Therapy, Respiratory Therapy, or Public Health Nursing. Full information about patients was not routinely made available to the team leader, who was unable to pass on the information to nurses on the next shift. This lack of dialogue resulted in an uncoordinated approach to patient care. Goals of patient care were not discussed; it was all too possible for a patient to have a remission goal, the doctor a research goal, and the nurse a terminal-care goal. Coordinating communication among the various departments was often left up to the patient, who would be asked by a doctor or nurse what was being done for him in Physical Therapy, say, or what point he had reached in a treatment program.

RECOMMENDATIONS

The researcher's recommendations from the conclusions derived from this study pertain to the care of cancer patients, the education of nurses, directions for change in the health care delivery system, and further research.

1. Greater emphasis should be placed on the affective component of educational programs for early detection of cancer. For example, such programs should address people's attitudes, feelings, and values about breast self-examination and smoking rather than just teaching facts and techniques.

2. Persons who care for the very sick and dying should not be required to function in a constant frenzy of activity so that they deny patients' requests to talk about their experiences and deny families the opportunity for group support in coping with the stresses. The family forms the matrix of existence for the dying person, and if families are given appropriate support, patients will benefit. If staff can learn to support patients and families, learn to understand the cause and meaning of patients' behavior (such as anger), and learn appropriate strategies for intervention, they will gain more satisfaction from their work. A realistic approach begins with providing sufficient staff so that they have time to give patients and families emotional support as well as meet physical and physiologic needs for care, although it is recognized that frenzied activity can be a way to avoid planning, avoid the feelings of patients, and avoid other aspects of ideal role performance. In addition, staff who work on oncology units must value, develop skill in, and be accountable for psychosociocultural aspects of care.

3. Physicians and members of supporting departments, as well as nursing staff, need help in dealing with the psychologic and sociocultural aspects of caring for cancer patients and in dealing with their own emotional responses.

4. Planned interdisciplinary dialogue, with input by patient and family, is essential to promote coordination of care.

5. The physical setting of an oncology unit should provide an area for patients and families to meet for group support as well as diversion. Patient access to a kitchenette would promote better nutrition.

6. All nursing units should provide private space for the nursing staff to relax, think, and plan, particularly the head nurse.

7. If a hospital is to meet its goals of patient care, it must sponsor and evaluate ongoing nursing inservice education programs that provide for growth in intellectual knowledge and emotional support processes as well as psychomotor skills.

8. There is an imperative need for nursing supervisors and inservice education staff to be prepared at the master's degree level in an appropriate field of clinical nursing specialization.

9. Measures of quality assurance of nursing care for hospitalized cancer patients should be developed and implemented by departments of nursing service.

10. Coordination of patient care is very complex because of advances in nursing science, increased technology, new diagnostic tests, the complexities of medical care and drug treatment, and the fragmentation of care by a large array of allied health workers. Many of the tasks currently performed by the head nurse and supervisor should be performed by a nonnurse unit manager so that the supervisor and head nurse can be free to coordinate patient care and supervise nursing staff instead of having to correct the deficiencies of other departments.

11. It is realistic to expect some nurses to leave the full-time practice of their profession temporarily because of marriage, child-rearing, or other personal choices. Therefore, continuing education for relicensure, under the control of the nursing profession, should be required. Refresher or return-to-nursing courses, which to date are frequently refresher programs in psychomotor skills, should be based on a resocialization model, with a goal of enhancing professional self-concept and emphasizing theoretical foundation for practice as well as skills.

12. Because of the societal traditions of male dominance and female passivity and the reinforcement of these values in the traditional education of physicians and nurses, assertiveness training for nurses should be emphasized in basic, inservice, and continuing education programs.

13. The tendency of nurse graduates of hospital and associate degree programs to seek degrees in nonnursing fields represents a loss to the individual and the profession, as well as to consumers. Colleges and universities, particularly those that are state sponsored, should seek quality-controlled means to facilitate the professional education of such graduates to increase their potential for full contribution to society. High school guidance counselors should guide potential nursing students initially to the associate degree or baccalaureate program that matches their potential. It is recognized that hospital schools of nursing are in a phasing-out period; and this movement should be continued. Those who counsel prospective nursing students have an ethical responsibility to advise them of the personal and professional risks involved in choosing a hospital school rather than a nursing program that is in the mainstream of American higher education. At the same time nurse educators who are

concerned with the professional socialization of neophytes should be wary of eliminating all that was included in hospital-based training without examining this system for its positive as well as its negative aspects.

14. Nurse educators should communicate more with service agency personnel and jointly plan to prepare nurses for the role transition from student to employee. Prospective hospital nursing staff should be given a realistic view of the problems and issues involved on particular nursing units.

15. Nurses employed in hospitals, particularly staff nurses, need to form a strong colleague reference group in order to effect change.

16. The physiologic and psychologic components of the care of cancer patients are a necessary part of the nursing curricula; however, educators should give comparable attention to the sociological factors in agencies that influence the role boundaries of nursing practice. Basic and continuing education programs should prepare the nurse to deal with subsystem constraints on effective nursing practice.

17. Nurses frequently implement medical orders that have ethical dimensions. An arena should be provided where doctors, nurses, and others involved can discuss these bioethical dilemmas in good faith.

18. The significance of the bioethical issues involved in informed consent, research protocols, and the prolongation of life, as well as the nurse's ideologic role as the patient's advocate, points out the need for increased emphasis on the study of ethics and the principles of clinical research in the basic and continuing education of nurses.

19. In hospital billing, the cost of nursing care is included in the basic daily rate. Thus it is impossible to determine from the per diem rate how much is allotted for nursing care and how much for hotel maintenance (bed and food) and other nonnursing costs, such as new technology, basic supplies, or general overhead. Nor is it possible to determine how much of the nursing allotment actually represents compensation by nurses for the inefficiencies of other hospital departments. These costs would be readily apparent if, for example, individual nurses contracted for their services with the hospital administration, or if a nursing service department severed itself from hospital administration and contracted with the hospital as a private corporation, supplying nursing services only. Alternatives to the present billing system should be studied so that the public and the professionals have a true assessment of the costs of nursing care for various intensities of illness.

20. The realities of the physical, intellectual, and emotional involvements of staff-level, hospital-based nursing practice, where the majority of nurses are currently employed, as well as the need for older women (often self-supporting) to be employed, suggests that the nursing profession should devote attention to the needs of its aging members.

21. This descriptive study demonstrates that care and cure are different but integral parts of a therapeutic process. In many other cultures, as Leininger notes, caring is a higher priority than curing, but American society places greater emphasis on cure, curing, and the cure-giver [8]. But caring is an important part of curing, and when cure is not possible, caring is the only thing. Caring is an important but neglected dimension of health maintenance, prevention of illness, restoration of health, and preparation for death. Other professionals and the public should become more aware of, supportive of, and value its nursing care-givers, not just its cure-givers. In the subculture studied, nursing staff received some positive feedback from patients and families on their caring behaviors. Unfortunately, the staff did not discuss or analyze these behaviors so that they could apply them to other situations.

RECOMMENDATIONS FOR FURTHER RESEARCH

This research has generated a wealth of ideas for further study, including the following.

1. Powerlessness of patients and nurses in a bureaucratic, service-oriented organization.

2. Comparison of cancer patients housed on oncology units and of those on mixed medical-surgical units of general hospitals.

3. Racism in hospitals and its effect on patient care.

4. Further studies of sexism in hospitals.

5. Personality studies of oncologists.

6. Personality studies of oncology nursing personnel.

7. Nurses' caring behaviors, that is, what deliberate, scientifically selected actions are identified as caring behaviors, as contrasted with sentimental behaviors.

8. Patients and families perceptions, staff's laughter and humor in "situation-limits" environments where grief, anxiety, anger, and the prospect of dying are commonplace.

9. Comparative studies of salaries of registered nurses, other hospital personnel, and physicians.

10. Incentive programs to make evening and night staff nursing more attractive.

11. Issues involved in employing aging nurses at the staff nurse level.

12. Ethnographic studies of other hospital subsystems, such as the Intensive Care Unit or Radiation Therapy Department.

13. Ritualistic behaviors of nurses.

14. Attitudes of physicians and nurses toward obese patients.

15. Problems common to hospitalized cancer patients such as the management of pain, diversion, nutrition, mouth lesions, skin breakdown, nosocomical infection, and gastrointestinal malfunction.

16. Further studies of dying in a hospital, particularly of patients perceived by physicians and nurses to be "difficult" dying patients.

17. Disguised communication indicating that a patient has reached the acceptance stage in the dying process.

18. Epidemiologic investigations of cancer in marital dyads.

Lastly, it is essential that nurse researchers, educators, administrators, and others in positions of leadership support the nursing staff who are in daily contact with cancer patients, for the patient is remote from those leaders who are attempting in their own ways to improve the system of health care delivery. Those who are caring for cancer patients in their daily lives need the support of the public and their colleagues at every level.

> *. . . . never send to know for whom the bell tolls; it tolls for thee.*
> *John Donne*

REFERENCES

1. Ashley, J. *Hospitals, Paternalism, and the Role of the Nurse.* New York: Teachers College Press, 1976, p. 128.
2. Grissum, M., and Spengler, C. *Womanpower and Health Care.* Boston: Little, Brown, 1976, pp. 166-167.
3. Sills, G. Nursing, medicine, and hospital administration. *Am. J. Nurs.,* 76: 1439, 1976.
4. Grissum, M., and Spengler, C. 1976, pp. 166-167.
5. Ashley, J. 1976, p. 128.
6. Sills, G. 1976, p. 1432.
7. Grissum, M., and Spengler, C., 1976, p. 39.
8. Leininger, M. Caring: The Essence and Central Focus of Nursing. Part V in *The Phenomenon of Caring.* American Nurses' Foundation Nursing Research Report, 12: 14, 1977.

Bibliography

Books

Alexander, E. *Nursing Administration in the Hospital Health Care System.* St. Louis: C. V. Mosby, 1972.

Alsop, S. *Stay of Execution: A Sort of Memoir.* Philadelphia: J. B. Lippincott Co., 1973.

Barrett, J., Gessner, B., and Phelps, C. *The Head Nurse* (3d ed.). New York: Appleton-Century-Crofts, 1975.

Bloom, S. *The Doctor and His Patient.* New York: Russell Sage Foundation, 1963.

Browning, M., and Lewis, E., (comps.) *The Dying Patient: A Nursing Perspective.* New York: American Journal of Nursing, 1972.

Coser, R. Some Social Functions of Laughter. In Skipper, J. and Leonard, R. (Eds.), *Social Interaction and Patient Care.* Philadelphia: Lippincott, 1965, pp. 292-306.

Davis, M., Kramer, M., and Strauss, A. *Nurses in Practice. A Perspective on Work Environments.* St. Louis: C. V. Mosby, 1975.

Illich, I. *Medical Nemesis.* London: Caldor and Boyars, 1975.

Jaco, E. H. (Ed.), *Patients, Physicians and Illness* (2d ed.). New York: Free Press, 1972.

Jacobs, G. Ed. *The Participant Observer: Encounter with Social Reality.* New York, George Braziller, 1970.

Kramer, M., and Schmalenberg, C. *Path to Biculturalism.* Wakefield, Mass.: Contemporary Publishing, 1977.

Kubler, Ross, E. *Death. The Final Stage of Growth.* Englewood Cliffs, N.J.: Prentice Hall, 1975.

Lohr, W. System Characteristics that Influence Behaviors. In J.W. Cullen, B.H. Fox, and R.N. Isom (Eds.), *Cancer: The Behavioral Dimensions.* New York: Raven Press, 1973, pp. 125-136.

Marram, G.D., Schlegel, M., and Beris, E. *Primary Nursing: A Model for Individualized Care.* St. Louis: C.V. Mosby, 1974.

Mayers, M., Norby, R., and Watson, A. *Quality Assurance for Patient Care: Nursing Perspectives.* New York: Appleton-Century-Crofts, 1977.

Merton, R. *Social Theory and Social Structure* (Enlarged ed.). New York: Free Press, 1968.

Mullan, F. *White Coat: Clenched Fist. The Political Education of an American Physician.* New York: Macmillan, 1976.

Parsons, T., et al. *Theories of Society.* (two vol. in one). New York: Free Press, 1961.

Paterson, J., and Zderad, L. *Humanistic Nursing.* New York: John Wiley & Sons, 1976.

Pattison, E.M. (Ed.), *The Experience of Dying.* Englewood Cliffs, N.J.: Prentice Hall, 1977.

Robinson, D. *Patients, Practitioners and Medical Care*. London: William Heinemann Medical Books, 1973.
Vollmer, H., and Mills, D. *Professionalization*. Englewood Cliffs, N.J.: Prentice Hall, 1966.

Articles

Alfano, G. Healing or caretaking—which will it be? *Nurs. Clin. N. Amer*. 6: 273-280, 1971.
American Nurses' Association. Collective bargaining: what is negotiable? *Am. J. Nurs*., 69: 1891-1896, 1969.
Bates, B. Doctor and nurse: changing roles and relations. *N. E. J. Med*. 283: 129-134, 1970.
Benoliel, J. Scholarship—a woman's perspective. *Image,* 7: 22-27, 1975.
Byerly, E. The nurse-researcher as participant-observer in a nursing setting. *Nurs. Res.*, 18 (3): 230-236, 1969.
Clemence, M. Existentialism: a philosophy of commitment. *Am. J. Nurs.*, 66: 500-505, 1966.
Davitz, L., and Davitz, J. How do nurses feel when patients suffer? *Am. J. Nurs.*, 75: 1505-1510, 1975.
Dunphy, J.E. Annual discourse—on caring for the patient with cancer. *N. E. J. Med.*, 313-319, 1976.
Ethical dilemmas in nursing. Special supplement. *Am. J. Nurs.*, 77: 845-876, 1977.
Galub, S., and Resnehoff, M. Attitudes toward death—comparison of nursing students and graduate nurses. *Nurs. Res.* 20: 503-508, 1971.
Gaynor, A., and Berry, R. Observations of a staff nurse: an organizational analysis. *J. Nurs. Admin*. 3 (3): 43-49, 1973.
Inagaki, J., Rodriguez, V., and Bodey, G. Causes of death in cancer patients. *Cancer,* 33: 568-573, 1974.
International Encyclopedia of the Social Sciences, Vol. 7 S.V. Humor.
Lewis, F. "The Nurse as Lackey: A Sociological Perspective." *Supervisor Nurse* 7: 24-27, 1976.
Menzres, I. A case study in the functioning of social systems as a defense against anxiety: a report on a study of the nursing service of a general hospital. *Human Relations,* 13: 95-121, 1960.
Murray, W.B., and Buckingham, R.W. (Eds.). Implications of participant observation in medical studies. Editorial in *Canad. Med. Assoc. J.,* 115: 1187-1190, 1976.
Parsell, S., and Tagliareni, E. Cancer patients help each other. *Am. J. Nurs.*, 74: 650-651, 1976.
Peplau, H. Professional closeness. *Nurs. Forum,* 8 (4): 344-359, 1969.
Ragucci, A. The ethnographic approach and nursing research. *Nurs. Res.* 21 (6): 485-490, 1972.
Rodgers, J. Theoretical considerations involved in the process of change. *Nurs. Forum,* 12 (2): 160-174, 1973.
Sonstegard, L., et al. The grieving nurse. *Am. J. Nurs.*, 76: 1490-1492, 1976.
Thomas, L. A meliorist view of disease and dying. *J. Med. Philos.,* 1 (3): 212-221, 1976.
Ujhely, G. "And" instead of "either-or" or the "fallacy of false opposition." *Image,* 4 (3): 10-13, 1970-71.

Unpublished Material

Galton, R. The "Nurse Clinician Coordinator": A Study of an Expanded Role for Nurses in Ambulatory Care. Ph.D. dissertation, Columbia University, 1974.

Index

Admissions, 60-61; emergency, 61
Aides, 36, 129-30, 139-41, 146, 158, 217; as team members, 139-42; fear of dying patients, 145; student, 138-39; wages, 37
Ambulatory patients, 47-48, 64, 66. *See also* Self-care patients
American Cancer Society, 79, 158, 160, 190
American Nurses' Association, 4, 37, 150, 212
Anthropology, in a hospital, 13-22
Antibiotic research, 105, 156
Ashley, 3, 215
Assertiveness training, 224
Attendants, 72-73, 75

Bedside manner, 86-87
Benoliel and Crowley, 9
Bioethical issues, 108, 160, 211, 225
Blood: vomiting, 63; transfusions, 62, 100
Bone scan, 75
Brain scan, 76, 83-84, 91
Breast cancer, 83, 102, 182
Bruyn, 17, 22
Byerly, 7, 12

Cachexia, 63, 185
Cancer: as chronic disease, 8, 9, 69; attitudes toward, 69-70; breast, 83, 102, 182; detection of, 182, 223; diagnosis of, 8, 10, 69, 86; gastrointestinal, 63; lung, *(See* Lung cancer); of the colon, 199, 204; of the ovary, 190-91; of the

testicle, 110; of the thyroid, 200; prevention of, 182; prognosis in, 10, 87, 100; rectal, 184, 192; using word, 160. *See also* Oncology
Cancer nursing, literature of, 9-10
Cancer patients, 181-89, 222-23; ambulatory, 9, 47-48, 64, 66; appearance of, 184-86; at home, 10, 190-91; boredom of, 64, 65; care of, 9; common problems of, 149; hospitalized, 8, 9, 149; needs of, 70. *See also* Patients
Cancer treatment, methods of, 8-9
Cancer ward, vs. "mixed" ward, 66, 67-69, 70, 80. *See also* Oncology unit
CAT (computerized axial tomography) scanner, 76
Chaplain, 52, 60, 188, 195
Charles Hospital (pseud.), 2, 13-17; administration of, 28-35, 211; and medically indigent patients, 31-32; financial management, 31-32; history of, 25-35; medical school affiliation, 31; Nursing Department, 35-45; School of Nursing, 16, 27-28, 35, 69, 114
Charts, 55, 56, 114-15
Chemotherapy, 70, 83, 115, 159, 185; hair loss after, 70, 87, 99, 185; intraspinal administration of, 87; intravenous, 114; response rate to, 86; side effects of, 186; vomiting after, 147, 188
"Coding", 110-11
Collective bargaining, 212-13. *See also* Unions

ment by, 91, 197, 199; statistics on,
181-82. *See also* Cancer patients
Pharmacy, 50, 56, 77, 104-5
Physician's assistant, 95, 117, 159
Prognosis, 10, 87, 100
Progress notes, 33-34, 58, 115
Psychiatric consultation, 83, 174
Public Health Nursing, 79-80

Quint, 11-12, 20

Racial issues, 166, 204, 207
Radiation therapy, 72-74, 78, 101,
112, 137; in lieu of surgery, 192;
reactions to, 146-47, 150, 207; side
effects of, 186
Reality shock, 4, 173-78. *See also*
Ideology-rality conflict
Registered nurses, 3, 40, 86, 210,
211, 213; compared with LPNs,
141-42, 145; on staff, 126-29, 221;
licensure of, 3-5, 126; role strain
of, 214-15, 221; wages, 37
Religion, role of, 130, 199, 202, 220
Research Committee, 105-6
Resuscitation, 109, 110-11
Rogers, Martha, 6
Roommates, 61, 66, 138, 142-43,
182, 187, 189; death of, 61, 197,
198
Rounds, 58, 82-90; "management",
29-30; nurses on, 116; patients'
view of, 98; timing of, 97-99

Self-care patients, 47-48, 69, 81. *See
also* Ambulatory patients

Septicemia, 63, 100, 102, 105
Shifts, 144-46, 212, 214
Social Service Department, 78
Standards of Nursing Practice, 43,
150-51
Standing orders, 62, 147, 149, 219
State health department, inspection
by, 131, 155-56
Steriods, 92-93, 113; Cushing's
syndrome and, 102, 113, 185

Team nursing, 126, 136-37, 151; conferences in, 146; conflicts in, 139-
41; leaders, 136, 137, 141-42, 144
Theft, problem of, 50, 79, 84, 179,
191
Therapy: occupational, 74; physical,
74; respiratory, 75; X-ray, 75. *See
also* Radiation therapy
Third-party payment, 104, 106, 111.
See also Medicare
Treatment: aggressive, 93, 99-100,
101, 102, 108, 109; nurses' attitudes toward, 99-102; philosophy
of, 76, 93, 96, 108-11, 222; refusal
of, 91, 101, 197, 199

Unions, 31, 36. *See also* Collective
bargaining

Visiting hours, 64-65
Volunteers, 130

Women's liberation movement, 8,
132, 211

X-ray department, 75-76